"In this book Dr Rachman and Dr Mattick bring to bear a lifetime of interest and training to a fine-edge understanding of what constitutes honest and authentic communication—especially in a therapeutic two-person context. With a clear vision of the difference between hypothesis, assumption, and axiom, the authors compare and contrast the therapeutic technique proposed by the classic psychoanalytic Freudian method with that of the empathic method proposed by Sandor Ferenczi in his 'Confusion of Tongues' discovery. The clinical case study of Freud's Dora is considered for discussion and analysis."

Henry Kellerman *is a psychologist, psychoanalyst, and author; his latest book is* The Psychoanalytic Codes: Encryption and Decryption

"Through the telescope of Ferenczi's 'Confusion of Tongues' and relying on their vast and deep knowledge of Ferenczi, Arnold Rachman and Paul Mattick painstakingly reanalyze Freud's treatment of Dora while demonstrating the chasm between Freud's and Ferenczi's respective approaches. As they outline Freud's theories and techniques, the authors provide an alternative Ferenczian/relational approach that is certain to stir meaningful heuristic controversy."

Robert J. Marshall *is a faculty at The Center for Modern Psychoanalytic Studies*

"Every one of us who has studied psychoanalysis has spent some time on Freud's 'Fragment of an Analysis of a Case of Hysteria,' better known as his Dora case. It remains, over a hundred years after its initial publication, a controversial piece. It retains its ability to excite passionate debate. You could say that it is a tribute to Freud that he persisted with its publication, containing as it does such clear errors and failure on his part.

You might think that over the intervening years the field of literature on the case has filled to overflowing and that no one of us could have anything new to say on it or any new perspective to bring to it. Not so. In this refreshing new contribution Drs Rachman and Mattick offer their thoughts on a re-reading of the Dora case from the point of view of the Confusion of Tongue's theory of Sandor Ferenczi.

What they offer is nothing short of a paradigm shift for psychoanalysis. Pointing out failings in Freud's Oedipal interpretations they propose a whole new way of working within the psychoanalytic framework.

They propose a way of understanding the experience of psychoanalytic psychotherapy which includes at its core the analytic relationship, transference and equally importantly, countertransference.

This small volume is a timely and welcome addition to the lexicon. It will be of interest to students and professionals within the field of psychoanalysis and beyond. It will be of particular interest to those tracking changes in the direction of the field towards a more relational perspective in keeping with the development of the Budapest School of thought."

Fergal Brady, *president, The Irish Psycho-Analytical Association*

Freud, Dora, and the Confusion of Tongues

Responding to growing interest in issues of gender and power as they arise within psychoanalysis, *Freud, Dora, and the Confusion of Tongues* reexamines Freud's iconic case of Dora from the perspective of Sandor Ferenczi's investigation of the sexual manipulation of children by adults.

Freud believed that his analysis of Dora demonstrated the truth of his Oedipal theory; his treatment was based on interpretations of her statements as evidence of an unresolved Oedipal conflict. In contrast, Ferenczi's Confusion of Tongues theory focused on the actual interactions between young people and adults who made use of their social status and power to substitute sexuality for the affection children desire. Where Freud located the origin of neurosis in psychological processes interior to the analysand, Ferenczi directed attention to the real traumatic aspects of the relationships between people. By such critical investigation, this book most strikingly shows that Freud's imposition of his interpretations on Dora, despite his sincere wish to be of help to her, represented an abusive retraumatization.

Arguing that it is essential to understand linguistic and other representational systems of experience, and the interrelation between the reproduction and transformation of self, in a contemporary analysis of Dora's case, this book will appeal to psychoanalysts, philosophers, and all those interested in a new understanding of classical psychoanalysis.

Arnold W. Rachman is a clinical psychologist and relational psychoanalyst who has contributed to the recovery of the life and work of Sandor Ferenczi and the Budapest School of Psychoanalysis.

Paul Mattick taught for many years at Adelphi University. He is author of *Social Knowledge* (1986), *Art in Its Time* (2003), and *Theory as Critique* (2018), among other books, articles, and reviews.

Psychoanalytic Inquiry Book Series
Joseph D. Lichtenberg
Series Editor

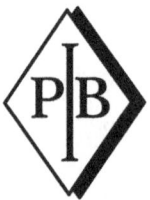

Like its counterpart, *Psychoanalytic Inquiry: A Topical Journal for Mental Health Professionals*, the Psychoanalytic Inquiry Book Series presents a diversity of subjects within a diversity of approaches to those subjects. Under the editorship of Joseph Lichtenberg, in collaboration with Melvin Bornstein and the editorial board of *Psychoanalytic Inquiry*, the volumes in this series strike a balance between research, theory, and clinical application. We are honored to have published the works of various innovators in psychoanalysis, including Frank Lachmann, James Fosshage, Robert Stolorow, Donna Orange, Louis Sander, Léon Wurmser, James Grotstein, Joseph Jones, Doris Brothers, Fredric Busch, and Joseph Lichtenberg, among others.

The series includes books and monographs on mainline psychoanalytic topics, such as sexuality, narcissism, trauma, homosexuality, jealousy, envy, and varied aspects of analytic process and technique. In our efforts to broaden the field of analytic interest, the series has incorporated and embraced innovative discoveries in infant research, self psychology, intersubjectivity, motivational systems, affects as process, responses to cancer, borderline states, contextualism, postmodernism, attachment research and theory, medication, and mentalization. As further investigations in psychoanalysis come to fruition, we seek to present them in readable, easily comprehensible writing.

After more than 25 years, the core vision of this series remains the investigation, analysis and discussion of developments on the cutting edge of the psychoanalytic field, inspired by a boundless spirit of inquiry. A full list of all the titles available in the *Psychoanalytic Inquiry* Book Series is available at www.routledge.com/Psychoanalytic-Inquiry-Book-Series/book-series/LEAPIBS.

Recent Books in the Series:

Freud, Dora, and the Confusion of Tongues
Arnold W. Rachman and Paul Mattick

Freud, Dora, and the Confusion of Tongues

Arnold W. Rachman and Paul Mattick

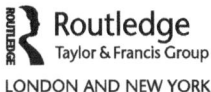
Routledge
Taylor & Francis Group

LONDON AND NEW YORK

First published 2023
by Routledge
4 Park Square, Milton Park, Abingdon, Oxon OX14 4RN

and by Routledge
605 Third Avenue, New York, NY 10158

*Routledge is an imprint of the Taylor & Francis Group, an informa
business*

British Library Cataloguing-in-Publication Data
A catalogue record for this book is available from the British
Library

Library of Congress Cataloging-in-Publication Data
Names: Rachman, Arnold W., author. | Mattick, Paul, 1944– author.
Title: Freud, Dora, and The confusion of tongues / Arnold W.
    Rachman, Paul Mattick.
Description: Abingdon, Oxon ; New York, NY : Routledge, 2023. |
    Includes bibliographical references and index.
Identifiers: LCCN 2022046537 (print) | LCCN 2022046538
    (ebook) | ISBN 9781032307718 (hardback) | ISBN
    9781032449531 (paperback) | ISBN 9781003306559 (ebook)
Subjects: LCSH: Psychoanalytic interpretation—Case studies. |
    Sex (Psychology)—Social aspects—Case studies. | Parent and
    child—Psychological aspects—Case studies. | Freud, Sigmund,
    1856–1939. | Bauer, Ida, 1882–1945. | Ferenczi, Sándor,
    1873–1933.
Classification: LCC RC509.8 .R334 2023 (print) | LCC RC509.8
    (ebook) | DDC 616.89/17—dc23/eng/20221122
LC record available at https://lccn.loc.gov/2022046537
LC ebook record available at https://lccn.loc.gov/2022046538

ISBN: 978-1-032-30771-8 (hbk)
ISBN: 978-1-032-44953-1 (pbk)
ISBN: 978-1-003-30655-9 (ebk)

DOI: 10.4324/9781003306559

Typeset in Times New Roman
by Apex CoVantage, LLC

Contents

Credits List

The authors gratefully acknowledge permission to republish the following material in this volume:

Extracts from *Three Essays on the Theory of Sexuality* by Sigmund Freud, copyright © 1976. Reprinted by permission of Basic Books, an imprint of Hachette Book Group, Inc.

Extracts from *Three Essays on the Theory of Sexuality*, ed. and trans. J. Strachey [New York: Basic Books, 1975]. By permission of The Marsh Agency Ltd., on behalf of Sigmund Freud Copyrights.

1 The Case of Dora

A Paradigm of the Confusion of Tongues

Freud's account of the failed analysis of the young woman he called "Dora" has become, during the last 30 years, the most discussed of his case histories. Some account for this by pointing to the recent increase of interest in issues of transference and countertransference in psychoanalysis, matters relevant to orthodox understandings of how Dora's treatment went awry.[1] It is obvious that another spur to reexamination of this case has been the rise of contemporary feminism and its academic wing's complex relation to psychoanalysis. The story of Freud and Dora, whatever else it is, is the story of a meeting, at the end of the nineteenth century, between a man armed with the power and authority of gender and the professional qualifications of a physician and a young girl struggling to maintain her integrity in the face of adult manipulations. The themes of gender, power, and the cultural imbrications of psychoanalysis have led to a widening of the flow of commentary to include writing by literary critics, historians, women's studies professionals, and even a linguist interested in the pragmatics of psychotherapeutic dialogue.[2]

The only valid reason for adding another item to this mass of commentary is the interest in a hitherto unexplored approach to the questions raised by Freud's text. What we believe we have to contribute emerged in the course of a joint reading of *Dora* by two people with very different interests and professional training. Arnold Rachman is a practicing psychoanalyst, with an interest in the nature of empathy, authenticity, and the curative function of the analytic relationship; he is particularly concerned with power, control, and status in that relationship. His ideas are informed by the Budapest School of psychoanalysis, particularly the contributions of Sándor Ferenczi and Michael Balint. Paul Mattick is a philosopher, with particular interests in linguistic and other systems for the representation of experience, and in the interrelations between the reproduction and transformation of social structure and individuals' construction of self.

DOI: 10.4324/9781003306559-1

What drew us together was a shared idea of experience as not given but shaped—within the constraints of social and interpersonal reality—by active subjects striving to maintain functional senses of self in the world. We wished at once to explore the consequences of this idea for the understanding and practice of psychotherapy and the contribution issues emerging in therapy might offer to the development of this idea. In the course of a discussion of one of Ferenczi's key contributions to the psychoanalytic literature, his paper, "The Confusion of Tongues Between Adults and Children," it occurred to us that Dora's experience with Freud could be understood in terms of the pathology of communication Ferenczi had identified in cases of the sexual abuse of children by adults. The more we read, thought, and discussed, the further this idea drew us into an investigation of psychoanalysis generally.

While many aspects of our critique of the practice of psychoanalysis are, we are happy to say, shared with other commentators on *Dora*, our approach is unique, so far as we know, in examining Freud's case study through the optic of Ferenczi's conception of the Confusion of Tongues. In this way, we have arrived at a critique of psychoanalysis from a starting point within it, for Ferenczi was a committed disciple of Freud and wished only to contribute to the further development of his master's method of thought and cure. The rejection of Ferenczi and his ideas by psychoanalytic orthodoxy, ironically, evinced a sensitivity to the depth of his critique that went beyond what Ferenczi himself could recognize. Lest it be thought that this rejection belongs entirely to the past, we note a recent response to our submission of a version of a chapter of this book to the *Psychoanalytic Quarterly*. Speaking for the editorial board, the editor wrote, quoting an editorial reader, that our text was

> basically a polemic for Ferenczi and a view of pathology and neurosis as an outgrowth of a "bad" parental environment. . . . [T]his type of reasoning that concludes that all of the trends in psychoanalysis which involve viewing it as a two-person psychology can be subsumed under the work of any early psychoanalyst, in his or her struggles with Freud, is misleading.
>
> The continuing attempt to treat Ferenczi as the heroic but tragically denied founder of contemporary psychoanalysis has had enough of an outing and opportunity in all too many papers and books. . . . It is a great mistake to leap-frog over the slow steps in progress to where we are today in order to elevate the work of any of our predecessors.

Whether this characterization of our text as primarily concerned with Ferenczi's importance is correct, the reader can ascertain by looking at the version of it included here as Chapter 4, which seems to us rather a critique of Freud. But might not this be closer to the point at issue? For the stricture in our critic's last sentence is hardly applied, in the pages of the *Psychoanalytic Quarterly* to the work of at least one of our predecessors.

Our intention is not to cast Ferenczi as a replacement for Freud as cult hero of psychoanalysis, although we find his theory of the Confusion of Tongues an invaluable starting point for reconceiving the analytic relationship. If we return to him periodically, and to his relations with Freud, in what follows, it is because, we feel, his attempts to rethink psychotherapeutic practice were fruitful and remain instructive.

One of us (AWR) has been accused by some in his profession of making Ferenczi into a hero and Freud into a villain. It is difficult not to want to give Ferenczi his place in the sun, after he was so unceremoniously relegated to the darkest corner of psychoanalytic history. The tendency to think of Ferenczi in heroic terms reflected the effort to rediscover and highlight the significant contributions to psychoanalysis as well as to encourage the use of him as a role model for contemporary clinical functioning. Indeed, Ferenczi's practice, it seems to us, represents an attempt to take the scientific aspect of Freud's theory more seriously than its inventor was able to do, by opening ways to alternative conceptualizations and experiments with clinical techniques. It also acknowledges the relational character of the psychoanalytic experience, with an insistence on the nature of the emotional relationship between analyst and analysand in place of Freud's sense of himself as scientist and his patient as an object of investigation. Ferenczi's alternative theory and method represents, we think, a more viable model for the treatment of emotional disorders in contemporary society.

The contemporary resilience of the Freudian viewpoint can be seen in Patrick Mahony's recent book, *Freud's Dora. A Psychoanalytic, Historical, and Textual Study*.[3] In this admirably scholarly work, in which Mahony, a practicing analyst, has labored to bring to light the historical truth of Dora's story, at the cost of exposing Freud on various important points as an outright fabricator, he also endorses the strongest feminist and related criticisms of Freud as a sexist power monger in his relations with his young patient. He speaks of the "dubiety" of Freud's "etiological explanations of Dora's trauma and symptoms, the tendentious and often reckless interpretations of her dreams, the absence of transferential interpretation, the failure to integrate Dora's gynecophilic strivings—her deepest psychic current—into the interpreted material."[4] But, as the inclusion of Dora's alleged homosexuality in this list suggests, Mahony at the same time credits Freud with teaching her "the history of her desire, which had left aches throughout her body in verbalizable meanings," even if they are only to be identified by "sifting through the sum of Freud's clinical biases, his unempathic relationship with

Dora, and his interpretive bullying and his forcing of her associations."[5] His critique of Freud's handling of the case assumes the fundamental correctness of the theory of which it is supposed to be an application.[6] Perhaps more startling is the hold of Freudian theory on feminist critics. Toril Moi, for instance, begins her essay on the Dora case by accusing Freud of being a sexist authoritarian, "a willing participant in the male power game conducted between Dora's father and Herr K." But she finds a deeper explanation for Freud's failure with Dora in Freudian terms: "Freud's countertransference blinds him to the possibility that Dora's hysteria may be due to the repression of desire, not for Herr K, but for his wife, Frau K." Thus Freud's "phallocentric epistemology" is undermined by means of "Freud's own theories of femininity and sexuality . . . We can only destroy the mythical and mystifying constructions of patriarchy by using its own weapons. We have no others."[7]

In fact, despite the mounting tide of criticism of Freud's methods and concepts brought by the last decades of the century that began with the publication of *The Interpretation of Dreams*, and despite the many alternate forms of psychotherapy that have been invented since Freud's time, Freudian theory remains the paradigm for practical and theoretical insight into the problems that bring people to therapists. This can be seen even in rather theoretically independent commentaries on the Dora case study. A striking example is the 1977 paper by Samuel Slipp, which uses the Dora case to propose a redefinition of hysteria in terms of interpersonal factors, specifically a pattern of family dynamics. In his discussion of Dora, whom he takes as a typical example of the hysteria syndrome, he nonetheless accepts Freud's imputation to her of sexual fantasies of various types: "Dora fantasized giving to her father and to Herr K what both their wives withheld from them, sex. . . . Dora enjoyed the sensual hothouse in which she lived. . . . [B]ecause of [an] identification with her father [she] manifested homosexual inclinations towards Frau K." While the theoretical framework is enlarged, the basic description of Dora's psychological state does not alter: "If we conceive of seduction as an interpersonal power maneuver and a style of relating to manipulate and control others instead of a unique sexual event," Slipp concludes, "Freud's original insights again become rich and meaningful."[8]

What accounts for this continuing dominance of Freudian thought? No doubt in part the obvious brilliance of Freud's conceptual construction, but also in part the near absence of alternative approaches matching Freud's generality and apparent explanatory power. It is due also to specific features of Freud's theory, which reflect both his wish to be a medical scientist and fundamental problems with the way in which he went about it.

For one thing, it combines descriptive complexity with analytic simplicity: All the interpretive sophistication of psychoanalysis rests on the foundation of a simple formula for human behavior. The superstructure of esoteric concepts reduces human behavior to the simplistic view that all its complexity derives from the individual's handling of sexual and aggressive drives. This viewpoint is a version of a conception of human nature deeply engrained in modern thought, stated clearly already in the seventeenth-century theorizing of philosophers like Hobbes and Locke: People are fundamentally self-seeking individuals, prodded into action by biological needs, the aggressive activity thus produced limited only by social constraints. This ideological conception takes on a biological coloring by way of the drive concept, and in this way seems a part of scientific medicine, however outmoded the concept of drive is at present.[9]

The putatively scientific status of the theory powers the analyst's insistence on the objective validity of his understanding of the analysand's troubles. If the individual doesn't accept the analyst's explanation of his or her behavior as a transformation of sexual and aggressive drives, this "resistance" is to be interpreted as confirmation; as Freud himself famously put it "No" means "Yes." The analyst keeps presenting his or her interpretation until the analysand accepts it, and deals with any objections to the analyst's behavior as part of the problem. It is true that in contemporary psychoanalysis insistence on resistance interpretations has given way to a more empathic approach. However, the goal of traditional analysis remains that of peeling away layers of resistance.

To go beyond this framework requires a more complicated, less formulaic view of human behavior, taking into account the vicissitudes of human interaction between individuals and groups. For instance, issues of power, control, and status have force of their own, not reducible to primitive energies of sex and aggression. Trauma is a structure of experience—or rather, a set of structures—to be understood in its own terms. The events that occur in relations between people, in all their complexity, cannot be reduced to symbols for a small set of fundamental factors. Ontological reduction is the counterpart of interpretive epistemology. Interpretation becomes the golden tool for understanding human behavior, because insufficient credence is given to the significance of actual events.

Of course, understanding is something other than the reproduction of experience; hence, the inevitability of principles of scientific thought on the model of Occam's Razor. While not the only criterion for satisfactory explanation, simplicity or conceptual parsimony is a desirable characteristic of explanatory frameworks. How is parsimony to be distinguished from reductionism? An example is furnished by Ferenczi's Confusion of

Tongues concept. As we will see, it provides a powerful explanatory device for an unfortunately large class of experiences, but it is not a general theory of the mind.

One alternative to reductionism is what we might call phenomenologically oriented understanding, where the analyst is attuned to an individual's attempts to inform him or her of their frame of reference, in contrast to interpreting their frame of reference. A famous incident in the course of Dora's treatment, to be discussed in greater detail below, provides an example. Having introduced the idea that Dora was a childhood masturbator, and that this was a contributing cause of her neurosis, Freud notices her playing with her reticule. He interprets this as a disguised form of masturbation and an implicit admission of the correctness of his diagnosis. A less reductive approach might have been to inquire as to Dora's own explanation of her action, trying to elicit in her words her own frame of reference for understanding her behavior. If she answered, for instance that she was anxious, Freud might have inquired why, rather than explaining her anxiety in terms of the psychogenetic history he has imagined for her.

Another form of oversimplification is Freud's tendency to examine relationships as if they were embodied in the individual in his office. This is in part because his theory stresses events it holds to occur within the individual psyche. But especially when psychotherapy takes the form of a one-on-one encounter, the analytic scope must be wide enough to take into account the reciprocal impact between individuals and the communities of people to whom they relate.

Further, in the therapeutic framework itself, analysts need to examine their own functioning. Part of Ferenczi's innovation was his discovery of the curative function of the analyst's contribution to the treatment process. His capacity to observe his own negative contribution to that process and to correct it, through analysis of his own attitudes, is a counter-model to Freud's mode of functioning in the Dora case. As we will emphasize repeatedly, Freud could not observe his own behavior as it contributed to the analytic encounter with Dora or—to give him credit for his powers of clinical observation—if he observed it he did not consider it primary. His focus was on analyzing Dora's purported Oedipal complex. In contrast, Ferenczi focused on analyzing the nature of the emotional relationships in his patients' lives as reflected in their relationships with him. Later analysts' reluctance to do this is the primary roadblock to advancing understanding and practice in the field of psychotherapy. To go beyond biology, we have to take seriously interpersonal and social dynamics both in the wider field of society and in the consulting room.

There is a hallowed tradition in science of the idea that the observer can contaminate the observation, and that guarding against this requires a sterile field of operations. In psychoanalysis—which in this regard has been very influential throughout the field of therapy—the analyst has been understood as ideally a detached observer. This element has been held onto even when other aspects of Freudian theory are dropped. Even interpersonalists, object-relations theorists, and self-psychologists, who pay homage to interpersonal aspects of the analytic experience, still maintain the idea that transparency of the analysis is not desirable, and it is not a part of the theory of the analytic encounter.

Arnold Rachman once submitted a paper on analysts' self-disclosure to a self-psychology conference. The first reaction to it of a senior, respected member of that community was, "You're not going to make us all reveal our faults!" Although the paper was accepted for publication and was well received by an audience of younger therapists and analysts, the senior clinicians and scholars were uniformly skeptical and critical of the very idea of self-disclosure. The self-psychological critique of this idea is that self-disclosure interferes with the subjective experience of the analysand and shifts the focus from the analyst's immersion in the subjective reality of the analysand. This is indeed the point at issue; from our point of view, this way of putting the question obscures the fact that subjective experience is shaped by an actual interaction between two people, and not only by the intrasubjective activity of the analysand.

Notes

1 See Jerry L. Jennings, "The Revival of 'Dora'," *Journal of the American Psychoanalytic Association* 34:3 (1986), pp. 607–635. Jennings also stresses the development of psychoanalytic theories of adolescence.

2 See, for example, Robin Tolmach Lakoff and James C. Coyne, *Father Knows Best: The Use and Abuse of Power in Freud's Case of Dora* (New York: Teachers College Press, 1993).

3 Patrick Mahony, *Freud's Dora: A Psychoanalytic, Historical, and Textual Study* (New Haven: Yale University Press, 1996).

4 Ibid., p. 146.

5 Ibid., pp. 145, 76.

6 Thus, Mahony suggests that "in treating Dora, Freud once more held at bay his own feminine identification and kept in suspense the enmeshed difficulties with transference and homosexuality that he had with Fliess" (pp. 46–47). He asserts, "Dora was beset by a torrent of unstable and contradictory identifications characterized by the displacements and condensations of preoedipal and oedipal elements" (p. 69).

7 Toril Moi, "Representations of Patriarchy: Sexuality and Epistemology in Freud's *Dora*," in *What Is a Woman? And Other Essays* (Oxford: Oxford University Press, 1999), pp. 330, 339, 347. For a similar inability to imagine an alternative source for what feminism needs to overcome the insufficiencies of social theory, despite the apparent inadequacy of Freud's understanding of women, see Muriel

Dimen, "Strange Hearts: On the Paradoxical Liaison Between Psychoanalysis and Feminism," in Michael S. Roth, ed., *Freud: Conflict and Culture* (New York: Alfred A. Knopf, 1998), p. 213.

8 Samuel Slipp, "Interpersonal Factors in Hysteria: Freud's Seduction Theory and the Case of Dora," *American Academy of Psychoanalysis* 5:3 (1977), pp. 359–376, 369, 370, 373.

9 A striking example of the hold on analytically oriented researchers of the idea of Freud as not only founder but master of his discipline is to be seen in John Bowlby's discussion of instinct and drive theory in *Attachment* (Harmondsworth: Penguin, 1971). While acknowledging that by accepting contemporary conceptions of instinct as organismic self-regulation "Freud's concept of *Trieb*, so unfortunately mistranslated as 'instinct,' is . . . dispensed with" (p. 217), he is still at pains to suggest that Freud would have been ready to give up his way of conceptualizing the problem (pp. 43–44).

2   The Confusion of Tongues

We are today familiar with the story of Freud's abandonment of his original "Seduction Theory" of neurosis for one that emphasized the primacy of analysands' fantasies of sexual relations with parental figures. Less familiar is the story of how Freud's favorite disciple, Sándor Ferenczi, came to propose a variation of Freud's original approach in a paper that he gave to the Twelfth International Psychoanalytic Congress at Wiesbaden, Germany on September 4, 1932. As Freud's leading student, his presentation had the coveted position as the opening address to the congress. However, it was received with extreme disapproval by the psychoanalysts present. Freud, prevented from attending because of the progression of his mouth cancer, also had a very negative reaction.[1]

Ferenczi came to his theory on the basis of 25 years of clinical work with what were called "difficult cases." His clinical career was based from the beginning upon individuals not treatable by traditional psychiatric means, people in the wards of the St Elizabeth and Rokus hospitals in Budapest who were criminals, prostitutes, homosexuals, and indigent people. His early clinical humanism was evident in one of his first reports.[2]

He asked "Rosa K.," imprisoned for transvestitism, to write an autobiography. By inviting her to explain her difficult life from her point of view, instead of assigning her to a diagnostic category and describing her life psychiatrically, he asked her to allow him to enter her subjective world. Thus he gave one of the first examples of an empathic method in psychotherapy. His clinical empathy also moved him to provide her with a letter, stating that her cross-dressing was a psychiatric and not a moral disorder, that prevented her from being rearrested.

When he discovered the work of Freud and met the man himself in 1908, their contact was a matter of immediate mutual attraction. Beyond the father–son dynamic that developed between the two, Ferenczi was excited by the power of Freud's ideas, while Freud was excited by Ferenczi's

DOI: 10.4324/9781003306559-2

clinical daring and emotional vitality. This led to a fruitful collaboration for a significant period of time. But Ferenczi's focus on "difficult cases" eventually led him to the development of a different approach from Freud's to the understanding of neurosis. These cases involved analysands who were not able to maintain the psychoanalytic paradigm of free association and interpretation. In response, Ferenczi invented a new mode of functioning for the analyst, who instead of an observer became an active partner in developing alternatives to free association. He began to detect a certain pattern in his "difficult cases." As he reported in his *Clinical Diary*,[3] it seemed clear that a majority of these people had been sexually molested as children, just as Freud had originally suggested in his Seduction Theory. But while Freud, theoretically ambitious and always ready to generalize from a few examples, had proposed his theory as an explanation for all neuroses, Ferenczi was reporting on a particular class of patients. His empathic listening led him to accept their accounts of childhood abuse as realities, not as symbolic Oedipal events. In this way, Ferenczi's empathy, a courageous choice of respect for the analysand's reality, challenged psychoanalytic orthodoxy.

Both his willingness to believe his analysands and his empathic and active clinical methods found full expression in his paper for the Twelfth Congress, "The Confusion of Tongues."[4] In this paper, Ferenczi addressed issues of trauma occurring in two realms of human behavior: the relation between parent and child, and the relationship between psychoanalyst and analysand. He drew a parallel between these two situations, suggesting the idea of retraumatization of the analysand in the therapeutic situation. This idea, of course, largely explains why this paper was so disturbing to the psychoanalytic community. Analysts of the time saw it as an indictment of themselves, particularly as they belonged to the upper-middle-class group in which Ferenczi had discovered child abuse. They felt accused in Ferenczi's paper of possible abuse both in their family relationships and in the clinical setting. And indeed, without intending to be confrontational, he was asking them to look at their clinical behavior as a function of their own personalities. He ushered in an evolutionary step: viewing the analytic encounter as a two-person experience.

Ferenczi addressed a number of significant issues in this paper: the deleterious effects of childhood sexual molestation on personality development, including such serious problems as dissociative disorders; a variety of defense mechanisms mobilized to cope with trauma; the fundamental psychodynamic of abusive relationship that he called "identification with the aggressor" (first described by Ferenczi and not, as generally thought, by Anna Freud)[5]; retraumatization in the psychoanalytic situation, an issue linked to what Ferenczi described as the "professional hypocrisy" of the analyst, whose interaction with the analysand is characterized by empathic failure; and a recommendation of analyst's self-disclosure as curative of such retraumatization experiences. The theoretical framework in which all these themes were developed he called "the Confusion of Tongues."

In his paper, Ferenczi reported on investigations into "the traumatic factor in the pathogenesis of neuroses" which had led him back to Freud's long-rejected "Seduction Theory." Using the more accurate term "rape," Ferenczi recounted that, when he was willing to give up his analytic presuppositions to listen to his analysands' explanations of their troubles, he discovered in their intractable emotional difficulties the aftereffects of severe emotional damage inflicted on them as children by adults. "Children," Ferenczi argued, may "play with the idea of taking the place of the parent of the same sex, in order to be the spouse of the opposite sex parent," as Freud's Oedipal theory claimed. But this is "only in fantasy; in reality they don't wish, indeed they are not able, to do without tenderness," which involves recognition of their special character and needs as children.

> If *more love*, or love of another sort than they wish, is forced upon children in the tenderness phase, this may have consequences quite as pathological as the *denial of love* that in the past has nearly always been brought up. . . . The consequences can only be that linguistic confusion to which I allude in the title of this lecture.[6]

In this way, Ferenczi stressed the structuring of trauma by confused communication. In an abusive relationship, parent and child speak different languages, even if they use the same words. The child speaks what Ferenczi called the language of tenderness and affection, demanding nurturance and love; the adult, desiring sexual experience, speaks the language of passion. While the child's expressed need for tenderness is appropriate, indeed necessary for development, the adult's desire for passion with a child represents a pathology, the developmental result of his or her own history of trauma.

Ferenczi speaks of confusion because the adult's behavior cannot make psychological sense to the child. Depending upon the child's pre-trauma personality development, family psychodynamics, and sociocultural experience, the child, even if he or she responds sexually, has an inherent sense that the adult's passion is not appropriate. (This, it should be noted, is an issue unaddressed by the Oedipal theory.) Neediness can move a child toward responsiveness, but the afterimage of confusion will persist: the child is left, emotionally and cognitively, with a sense of confusion about what has transpired with the adult, knowing at some level that passion is not affection but at the same time wishing to accept the abuser's definition of the event. The adult is also in a state of confusion, unable to distinguish between his or her aggressive, self-serving need for passion and the tenderness for which the child really longs. The child's use of identification with the aggressor as a mechanism of psychological defense intensifies the confusion, as identifying with the aggressor helps the victim maintain the fiction that the experience was one of tenderness.

An adult's passion for a child is not tenderness, it is sexuality—implicit and explicit expression of desire for erotic contact—even though the adult tries to maintain the fiction that it is tenderness, and tries to convince the child it is in the latter's best interest. The Freudian theory of infantile sexuality thinks of the child as itself having sexual wishes directed toward the parent. It is quite understandable, therefore, that Ferenczi's ideas were disturbing to Freud and the Freudians. As we will see, Freud could not believe that Dora at 14 did not welcome the sexual advances of the 40-year-old man who molested her. From the Ferenczian point of view, sexual contact between parent and child disrupts the intrapsychic fantasy process. The seduction intrudes upon the child's developmental need for a fantasized romance with the adult. If there is such a fantasy, the child should be allowed to have it without it becoming a reality.

Ferenczi was attempting to explicate the differences in language, behavior, and feeling arising between children and adults in an abusive experience. From his point of view, what parades as tenderness is clearly aggression. Such aggression is verifiable, since molestation is usually combined with physical threats. The child is told, for instance, that mentioning the abuse will be punished with physical harm. What is even more alarming, and intensifies the state of confusion, is that the parent may also threaten to withhold love if the act of violation is mentioned. The relational complexity involves the natural power a parent can exercise over a child. An abusing parent intensifies this issue by deliberately using unequal status to give expression to his or her narcissism and sadism.

The child has developmentally become accustomed to expect tenderness and affection in the form of emotional and physical nurturance of a nonsexual nature. A child wants and should receive tenderness and not sexual passion. A distinction between physical touch as affection and touch as sexuality must be made. We can think of this distinction as one between the adult's motivation to fulfill the child's need for affection and a self-centered gratification of the adult. In this situation, sexuality and power are closely connected. We are, after all, talking about a form of rape, the use of sexual activity to assert superior force in an interpersonal situation.

A child, because of his or her developmental need for parental affection, is emotionally prepared to yield to an adult. The emotional and interpersonal bargain is: I will give you the sex you want because I need the affection or love you will give me. Fundamentally, at the deepest level of the child's experience, although he or she does not speak of the act, the seduction is "a rape of the body and soul."[7] Psychological wounds persist long after the abuse has terminated.

As the child is traumatized by intrusion, aggression, and betrayal, a sense of confusion leads to a suppression of language. Speech is inhibited by fear and anxiety, concern about betraying one parent to another, threats of violence or withdrawal of love, the complicity of the non-abusing parent, the child's own psychopathology, and the feeling that he or she will be labeled a "hysterical liar." Often the victim is blamed in sexual incidents because no one wishes to confront the reality of evil in his or her spouse, friend, neighbor, cleric, or teacher, as well as be forced to take action that may compromise the tenuous emotional and interpersonal equilibrium that has been established. *Unable to speak of the trauma, the child becomes tongue-tied.* The adult seducer also does not speak of the seduction. In Jeffrey Masson's words, "the guilt that the parent or parental surrogate ought to feel but does not is then introjected by the child (the act is perceived as wrong, but there is no one else to take responsibility for it except the child victim)."[8]

The child, in order to cope with the trauma—that is, maintain self-cohesion and affectionate ties to the parent, and continue interpersonal contact necessary for survival—develops a series of defense or coping measures. One could also label them "trauma survival measures," that is, intrapsychic and interpersonal and intellectual measures to reduce the sting of the emotional crisis that threatens to overwhelm the individual.

Ferenczi was the first to describe the pathogenic defense mechanism "identification with the aggressor" as a means of coping with trauma: if

> the same anxiety . . . reaches a certain maximum, [it] compels [seduced children] to subordinate themselves like automata to the will of the aggressor, to divine each one of his desires and to gratify these; completely oblivious of themselves, they identify themselves with the aggressor.[9]

This mechanism can aid our understanding of the psychodynamics of victimization. A child who has been abused by an adult internalizes a sense of victimization by virtue of his or her sense of physical and emotional helplessness. If this dynamic is not worked through in childhood or adolescence, the individual enters adulthood "programmed," as it were, to repeat the experience of being a victim either to perceived abuse or by recreating the experience of abuse. Identification with the aggressor can also explain the phenomenon of a child acting out sexual abuse. An abused child can become preoccupied with sexual matters, for instance, in the form of precocious sexuality lacing verbal or physical behavior. Such a child may subsequently molest a sibling or friend. (This phenomenon aids in the understanding of the persistence of abusive behavior in the second, third, fourth, and even fifth generations of families.)

Does the child make himself accept the adult's point of view or does it pretend to do so? Through the mechanism of the identification with the aggressor, the child loses full contact with reality, accepting the abuser's definition of reality, in order to maintain the fiction of affection and tenderness. The result is that the child becomes susceptible to an adult or authority defining their reality through the evocation of superior power, control, and status.

At the same time, the apparatus of "repression"—identification with the aggressor, dissociation, etc.—has the function of preserving self-cohesion. The sense of self becomes an internally complex one, as the child strives to combine acceptance of the adult point of view with the maintenance of his or her own point of view; the experience of self is accordingly one of conflicting constructions of interpersonal reality. In this way, the child organizes the idiosyncratic elements of personality around the traumatic events.

Although Ferenczi developed the concept of the Confusion of Tongues in relation to the sexual abuse of children, he generalized the experience to the psychoanalytic situation, discussing the effects that the analyst's power could have in imposing his worldview on the experience of an analysand.

> Gradually, then, I came to the conclusion that the patients have an exceedingly refined sensitivity for the wishes, tendencies, whims, sympathies and antipathies of their analyst, even if the analyst is completely unaware of this sensitivity. Instead of contradicting the analyst or accusing him of errors and blindness, the patients *identify themselves with him*; only in rare moments of an hysteroid excitement, i.e. in an almost unconscious state, can they pluck up enough courage to make a protest; normally they do not allow themselves to criticize us, such a criticism does not even become conscious in them unless we give them special permission or even encouragement to be so bold.

Ferenczi went on to specify how the traditional analytic encounter encourages an emotional trauma between analyst and analysand:

> The analytical situation—i.e. the restrained coolness, the professional hypocrisy and—hidden behind it but never revealed—a dislike of the patient which, nevertheless, he felt in all his being—such a situation was not essentially different from that which in his childhood had led to the illness. When, in addition to the strain caused by this analytical situation, we imposed on the patient the further burden of reproducing

the original trauma, we created a situation that was indeed unbearable. Small wonder that our effort produced no better results than the original trauma.[10]

More generally, sexual seduction can be seen as a special case of a psychodynamic characterized by empathic failure, leading to emotional rejection, abandonment, and deprivation: An authority causes an emotional disturbance, which can be conceptualized as an empathic break, in his or her relationship with another person (a child, adolescent, or adult). Aware of this disturbance, the other person attempts to engage in some form of dialogue about it. The authority figure, however, reacts by doing several further disturbing things, such as disavowing causing or contributing to the break; blaming it on the other person; and failing to contribute to a repair of the break. This behavior can lead the other to become confused and question his or her version of the disturbance, accepting the authority's definition of reality. If this kind of empathic disturbance is consistent in the relationship, the other may employ pathological mechanisms to adapt to the trauma.

Speaking in conflicting languages, dealing in miscommunication, practicing double-bind messages, and enacting differences in status and power by way of behavior are indications of the Confusion of Tongues. For example, a child says to a parent, "Why are you angry at me?" And the parent replies, "I'm not angry at you. I'm just trying to point out that ...." The child has sensed something in the adult's habitus that indicates displeasure. The parent denies having negative feeling or having expressed negative behavior. The child is left in a confused state ("I could have sworn my mother is angry at me, but she tells me she's not; I don't understand what's going on. Is there something wrong with me?"). The basic phenomenon is that the more powerful person in a dyad does not respond to the other person's view (wishes and feelings) about what is going on between them.

Ferenczi's introduction of the method of clinical empathy into psychoanalysis, correlatively, was an attempt to overcome the deleterious effects of differences in status and power between "physician" and "patient," and so to aid in overcoming the traumas suffered in earlier life.[11] In contrast to such a mode of procedure, as we shall see, Freud attempted to convince Dora of his worldview by repeated vigorous insistence that her emotional difficulties stemmed from her Oedipus complex. He paid no attention to her indications that she was suffering from what one might call the opposite emotional issue, a need for maternal tenderness and affection. The basic issue we wish to address is not whether he or she was "right" about her problems, but the nature of the communication between them. As we see it, it was an example of the Confusion of Tongues.

Notes

1 For a full account, see A.W. Rachman, *Sándor Ferenczi: The Psychotherapist of Tenderness and Passion* (Northvale, NJ: Jason Aronson, 1997).
2 Sándor Ferenczi, "Homosexualatus feminina [Female Homosexuality]," *Gyögyaszat* 11:167–168 (1902).
3 Sándor Ferenczi, *The Clinical Diary of Sándor Ferenczi*, ed. J. Dupont, trans. M. Balint and N.Z. Jackson (Cambridge: Harvard University Press, 1995 [1932]).
4 Sándor Ferenczi, "The Confusion of Tongues Between Adults and Children: The Language of Tenderness and Passion," in M. Balint, ed., *Final Contributions to the Problems and Methods of Psycho-Analysis*, vol. III (New York: Bruner/Mazel, 1980), pp. 156–167.
5 See J.M. Masson, *The Assault on Truth: Freud's Suppression of the Seduction Theory* (New York: Farrar, Strauss & Giroux, 1984); A.W. Rachman, *Sándor Ferenxzi*.
6 Sándor Ferenczi, "The Confusion of Tongues Between Adults and Children," p. 12.
7 We employ the words of L. Shengold, *Soul Murder* (New Haven: Yale University Press, 1989).
8 J.M. Masson, *The Assault on Truth*, pp. 148–149.
9 Sándor Ferenczi, "The Confusion of Tongues Between Adults and Children," p. 162.
10 Ibid., pp. 157–160.
11 See Sándor Ferenczi, "The Elasticity of Psychoanalytic Technique," in M. Balint, ed., *Final Contributions to the Problems and Methods of Psycho-Analysis*, vol. III (New York: Bruner/Mazel, 1980), pp. 87–102.

3   The Confusion of Tongues in Psychoanalysis

Freud and Ferenczi

A Confusion of Tongues experience requires understanding in terms of what we may call a two-person psychology. Ferenczi's original formulation specified the two parties as the abusing parent and the child victim. But one can extend this clinical paradigm to include the functioning of any authority figure with a subordinate, or more clearly stated, any relationship where there is an imbalance of status, power, and control.

They can be applied, interestingly, to the relationship between Freud and Ferenczi within which the concept of the Confusion of Tongues emerged. The analytic and personal relations between these two were marked by trauma, confusion, and double-bind communication. The understanding of the relationship between these two giants of psychoanalysis generally favors Freud. Ferenczi is typically described as an emotionally immature, dependent, ambivalent, and neurotic individual who demonstrated disturbed relationships with Freud and others.[1] There is a host of commentaries on the link between Ferenczi's neurotic personality (sometimes even seen as psychotic, as in the account in the final volume of Jones's Freud biography) and the development of his humanistic approach.[2] Why has there been a relative silence about Freud's neurotic personality and the link between his personality and the development of his clinical approach? In particular, why isn't Freud's behavior placed under the same scrutiny that Ferenczi has endured when the relationship between the two is discussed? One of us has suggested that traditional psychoanalysis, which has dominated the discourse about Freud the man, has practiced the phenomenon of *Todschweigen*, Death by Silence.[3] Traditional psychoanalysis has *silenced* scholarship and research on issues that threaten the Freud mystique, the view of Freud as an exemplar of personal and professional functioning. What is more, the practice of *Todschweigen* views dissidents who threaten this traditional view as unacceptable to mainstream psychoanalysis. The practice of *Todschweigen*

DOI: 10.4324/9781003306559-3

was originally developed to silence such dissidents as Adler, Jung, Rank, and Ferenczi, as when the latter's paper on the Confusion of Tongues was not published in English, as Jones had promised it would be.

This behavior can be compared to an abusive adult's injunction to an abused child not to speak of what has happened. This silencing is itself a further abuse, an attempt to block the mobilization of psychic (and social) resources to deal with traumatic experience. In Dora's story, as we shall see, the same pattern appears in Freud's insistence on an Oedipal interpretation of Dora's problems, an attempt to silence her expression of a need for parental tenderness.

In lifting the injunction on the practice of *Todschweigen* in discussing the Freud–Ferenczi relationship, we need to discuss the contributions of both men to their confusion of tongues. Freud acted neurotically in several instances. On the now famous trip the two took to Sicily in 1910, Freud's behavior in reality was quite different from the authorized version of the story told in the Jones biography and approved by Anna Freud as representative of the Freud family.[4] According to Phyllis Grosskurth's account, Freud may have led Ferenczi to believe that they would spend a portion of their vacation in Sicily writing a joint paper.[5] Ferenczi was ecstatic about the prospect of collaborating with the master. However, Freud's message about this collaboration was a confused one. When Ferenczi entered Freud's room to begin their joint work, Freud asked him to take dictation on the Schreber case, sending the message, "We are not co-authors; I am your superior." Ferenczi became angry and stormed out of the room.

One could view Ferenczi's behavior as neurotic, in that his anger and departure from the scene did not help resolve their differences, perhaps indicating that at this early point in the relationship he could neither create a more equal role with his mentor nor accept that his mentor did not want him as a peer. Freud clearly contributed to this difficulty through the mixed emotional messages he offered to Ferenczi. He disguised the language of authority as the language of collaboration. This was the Confusion of Tongues, a dynamic made possible because of Freud's actual dominance (like that of adult over child) in relation to Ferenczi. Ferenczi wanted mutuality but was offered subordination. Was Ferenczi's expectation of mutuality neurotic? Everything that has been written about the relationship during this initial phase suggests the existence of an affectionate, warm, collaborative relationship between them, something acknowledged in Freud's obituary for Ferenczi (and corroborated by Jones).

Freud wanted a particular kind of relationship with any colleague. Although he was friendly, responsive, and encouraging, he always wanted to retain the role of the Master. Ferenczi, like Jung before him, could never accept this limitation in their relationship. Freud struggled with the issue of mutuality but could not bend in this direction; perhaps he never recovered fully from the feeling that Wilhelm Fliess had betrayed their relationship, and never again allowed himself to be completely open to a colleague.

Erich Fromm's study of Freud's authoritarianism, *Sigmund Freud's Mission*, suggests that Freud played the role of an infallible leader.[6] He surrounded himself, as in the group of close followers called the Society of Rings, with what Fromm called "company men," the most dramatic example of which was Ernest Jones. Jones was totally devoted to Freud as a person and as the founder of psychoanalysis. It was he who suggested the formation of the Society of Rings to protect Freud and the psychoanalytic community from criticism from the outside. It is this kind of thinking, of us and them, that Freud embraced, if not initiated himself. It created the notion of a movement (more than a science) which must be protected from criticism and dissidence. Freud never lost the notion of being an embattled pioneer, a political leader who needed to protect his movement, continuing to fight the battle even though it had long been won.

It is this sort of parochial thinking and functioning that Freud applied to Ferenczi's dissident voice. Ferenczi took seriously the notion of psychoanalysis as a science, which needed to be open to revision of its ideas and methods on the basis of clinical experience. What is more, he took it seriously as a method of treatment, aiming at the relief of pain and therefore requiring above all responsiveness to the experience of analysands. Ferenczi had no political ambitions, turning down the presidency of the International Psychoanalytical Association to concentrate on the development of his theory and method of curing trauma.

It is this background of authoritarianism, parochialism, and orthodoxy that led Freud to conclude erroneously that Ferenczi was trying to break away from his mentor and leave the fold of mainstream psychoanalysis. Freud can be seen as "paranoid" in his belief that Ferenczi's Confusion of Tongues theory and the clinical experimentation with Relaxation Therapy were attempts to form his own school of psychoanalysis. In fact, Ferenczi never intended to break away from Freud (though Clara Thompson, for one, believed he should have done so). The difference between the two men was not, so to speak, institutional, but a matter of practical orientation. By Freud's own admission, he could not be the "mother in the transference," nor could he work in the zone of regression[7] or tolerate the emotional vicissitudes of the kind of "difficult cases" Ferenczi worked with. He did not see himself primarily as a healer[8]; his motivation was to build a comprehensive theory of human behavior and to establish that theory—psychoanalysis—as the foundation of scientific psychology. Ferenczi's primary motivation, in contrast, was to extend the boundaries of psychoanalytic therapy to include the treatment of trauma.

Freud did not understand the meaning of dissidence in science—that it aids the development of science. He believed that loyalty and conformity to the standard procedure were paramount. Ferenczi came within a hair's breadth of being expelled from the psychoanalytic fold. Freud could not embrace a loving son who wanted to examine and change his theory or method. In the terms of his own theory, Freud had an Oedipal problem with Ferenczi (as Ferenczi did with Freud). Freud did not let the son challenge the father, in order to find his own sense of self. Ferenczi, for his part, could not break away from Freud to give full expression to his ideas and clinical methods. He needed the constant approval of the father.

Freud could neither accept nor understand Ferenczi's clinical experimentation with difficult cases as an expression of Ferenczi's clinical genius or his passion (both neurotic and visionary) to heal emotional disorder and the traumas of incest. Thus, Freud sexualized Ferenczi's clinical experimentation with trauma survivors. When he heard through the grapevine that Clara Thompson boasted, "I can kiss Papa Ferenczi anytime I want," Freud assumed that Ferenczi was having sexual contact with his analysands. After hearing of Thompson's remark, Freud wrote Ferenczi what has become known as the "kissing letter" on December 13, 1931:

> I see that differences between us come to a head in a technical detail. . . . You have not made a secret of the fact that you kiss your patients and let them kiss you. . . . Why stop at a kiss? Which after all does not make a baby. And then bolder ones will come along, which will go further to peeping and showing . . . and petting parties . . . The younger of our colleagues will find it hard to stop at the point they originally intended, and God the Father Ferenczi, gazing at the lively scene he has created, will perhaps say to himself: Maybe after all I should have halted in my technique of motherly affection *before* the kiss.[9]

Ferenczi was wounded by the accusation of sexual acting out. He replied to Freud on December 27, in an unpublished letter Masson discovered at Maresfield Gardens on Freud's desk:

> I consider your fear that I will develop into a second Stekel unfounded [Stekel was noted for a tendency to invent case histories; he resigned from the psychoanalytic society in 1912, to Freud's evident relief.] The sins of youth, misdemeanors, if they are overcome and analytically worked through, can make a man wiser and more cautious than people who never even went through such storms . . . Now, I believe, I am capable of creating a mild, passion-free atmosphere, suitable for bringing forth even that which has been previously hidden.[10]

The basis for Freud's suspicion, beyond Clara Thompson's remark, was the "Elma affair." Ferenczi fell in love with Elma Palos after he began her analysis. She had come to him on the advice of her mother, Gisela, who was Ferenczi's mistress. (This was at a time when therapeutic boundaries were not yet in place.) The letters Ferenczi wrote to Freud during the time of her analysis with him reveal a mutual romantic interest. But careful investigation of the letters indicates no sexual contact between them. Ferenczi ended his romantic involvement, and Elma left the analysis. Ferenczi sent Elma to Freud for analysis; Freud used his knowledge of Ferenczi's romantic interest in her to damn the younger man's experiments with "relaxation therapy."

By 1932, Ferenczi had been a practicing analyst for 20 years, without any sexual incident with an analysand. In fact, sexual acting out is ruled out by the theory of trauma Ferenczi proposed in the Confusion of Tongues paper. Seductive behavior on the part of an analyst, even if unintentional, would be a retraumatization of the analysand. Ferenczi's letter indicates that he had analytically worked through his erotic feelings for Elma, someone he had wanted to marry, in order to maintain a therapeutic contact with her. The Elma affair may in this way have made a contribution to the understanding of the Confusion of Tongues, for Ferenczi in formulating a theory of sexual trauma was integrating his own clinical and professional experiences.

Ferenczi's willingness to practice "therapeutic touch" was fueled not by unresolved neurotic need to have physical contact with analysands but rather by a realization that incest survivors suffer from severe physical and emotional deprivation. In certain select instances, such as Thompson's, he experimented with physical contact as a contribution to the curative process. As Judith Dupont has observed, Freud misunderstood Ferenczi's behavior: "Contrary to rumor, Ferenczi did not kiss his patients. The story is based on a misunderstanding between Ferenczi and Freud, created by one of Ferenczi's patients (Clara Thompson) and which his clinical diary clarifies."[11] (It is worth noting that a colleague who had ongoing contact with Thompson while she was in analysis with Ferenczi reported that his clinical work with her produced significant positive results.)[12]

Ferenczi certainly seems to have gone beyond the bounds of therapeutic affection in the case of Elma, allowing himself to engage in a romantic crush, no doubt with sexual overtones. Freud's insistence that Ferenczi had actually had sexual intercourse with Elma, however, suggests a phantasy of the master's. It is as if Freud thought that, just as only the threat of castration held the libidinous infant from leaping upon his mother, so only the scientific coldness and distance of the analyst could prevent the transformation of the analytic couch into a bed of passion. Similarly, in his analysis of Dora, Freud suggests at one point that giving in to her need for affection would be tantamount to acting out sexually. This is a general fallacy of Freud's interpretive Oedipal theory: where there's love there's sex.

Freud assumed the position of the all-knowing father with Dora—as he was to do with Ferenczi—and he interpreted many if not all of her symptoms as manifestations of his version of parent–child conflict. Dora's difficulty, as Freud saw it, was based on her inability to resolve her sexual feelings toward her father. Freud virtually ignored her emotional problems with her mother. He attempted to forcibly convince Dora of the correctness of his version of her psychological experience, and he offered that as curative. He was also unmoved by the lack of potency of his own interpretations, which were not persuasive to Dora. He seems to be quite uninterested in what the other person has to say, in this way engaging in an "abusive dialogue," like that of a parent forcing his interpretation on a child for his benefit, not the child's.

In a peer relationship, as with Ferenczi, he did the same thing. Freud was ever the parent, the other the child. On the Sicily trip, he forced Ferenczi to be his secretary rather than collaborate, and when Ferenczi balked at this inequality he labeled him a neurotic child. Similarly, he forced his sexual interpretations on Dora and when she balked he labeled her an unanalyzable neurotic. In both these cases, the other person resisted Freud's attempt to define the relationship to a significant degree. Ferenczi, despite his enormous regard for Freud, never entirely gave in; Dora, although she came back to continue her analysis—thus showing that something in Freud's approach seemed promising to her—did not accept his mastery over their dialogue. Finding this unacceptable, Freud rejected her. In both instances, Freud had lingering doubts. He wondered, in his case history, if a different approach to Dora might have produced a different outcome. And after Ferenczi's death, Freud was able to acknowledge the other man as a peer. In his obituary for his student, he said, "He made students of us all."[13]

Sexuality as Analytic Construction

Aside from the immediate personal issues of the relationship between Ferenczi and Freud, the former's ideas raise important questions about the very foundations of Freudian theory. The concept of a Confusion of Tongues was developed to understand such a situation as that in which a parent is, for his or her own reasons, confusing a child's request for affection with a demand for sexual satisfaction. This conceptualization of such encounters suggests the need for a reevaluation of the psychoanalytic concept of infantile sexuality, which may itself represent the imposition of adult preoccupations on children's experience. It could even be argued that the most dramatic and widespread example of the Confusion of Tongues phenomenon is modern culture's bringing together of a wide variety of behavior by children and adults under the heading of "sexuality." In Michel Foucault's words, "Surely no other type of society has ever accumulated . . . a similar quantity of discourses concerned with sex." But this is not just a matter of talking more freely about a hitherto hidden phenomenon:

> In actual fact, what was involved, rather, was the very production of sexuality. Sexuality must not be thought of as a kind of natural given which power tries to hold in check, or as an obscure domain which knowledge tries gradually to uncover. It is the name that can be given to a historical construct.[14]

One of the chief points in social life at which that construct especially made itself felt was, again according to Foucault, the sexuality of children, especially as evidenced in masturbation.

Foucault considered that psychoanalysis played a key role in what he calls the "deployment of sexuality." Arguing along related lines, Arnold Davidson has emphasized that sexuality as a human attribute distinct from anatomy (where it was in general located before the late nineteenth century) "only became a possible object of psychological investigation, theorizing, and speculation because of a distinctive form of reasoning that had a historically specific origin" in the second half of the 1890s, what he calls "the psychiatric style of reasoning," the medicalization of a range of previously nonmedical moral, social, and physiological matters now analyzed in terms of such concepts as "impulses, tastes, aptitudes, satisfactions, and psychic traits" treated as definitive of essential types of person.[15]

In *Three Essays on the Theory of Sexuality* (1905), Freud insists that children are to be understood as explicitly sexual beings, in view of their oral, anal, and genital experiences.[16] Indeed, he claims that the whole surface of the body, and every internal organ, are potentially erogenous zones, that is, capable of sexual response. Thus, an infant suckling at the mother's breast is not just feeding, enjoying the sensation, and engaging in some sort of emotional contact, but exhibiting specifically sexual arousal. This is the beginning of infantile sexuality, in Freud's view: the infant discovers that the mouth is a source of pleasure. It is noteworthy that Freud makes no mention of the relational and affectionate component of the suckling experience; but then this is missing from the picture he gives of adult sex also, described fundamentally as the satisfaction of individual libidinal needs. For Freud, sex is not a relational experience but a drive reduction within the individual. This is how he can insist that sexual feeling is "independent of the object," transferable (in later life, in the perversions) to a material, an animal, or oneself. It is only the terror of castration that restricts the object of desire to the world of socially acceptable relationships.

This conception of sexuality pictures the sexual abuse of children by adults as the interaction, however unfortunate, improper, or even damaging to the child, between two sexually desirous beings. The sexual excitability of children "seduced" by adults, according to Freud, "shows that an aptitude for [all kinds of sexual irregularities] is innately present in their disposition." Freud invokes a venerable comparison, between children and working-class women: "In this respect children behave in the same kind of way as an average uncultivated woman in whom the same polymorphously perverse disposition persists."[17] It is hardly surprising that "the parents' affection for their child may awaken his sexual instinct prematurely," since children "themselves behave from an early age as though their dependence on the people looking after them were in the nature of sexual love."[18]

Instead of saying that Freud "discovered" infantile sexuality, one can say that he imputed sexuality to infants, thinking of it as similar to adult sexuality, although not necessarily located in the genitals. Classical psychoanalysis itself, that is, may be suffering from a confusion of tongues, in its application of a vocabulary developed for the analysis of adults to the understanding of children and adolescents, and in general misconstruing the expression of tenderness as an expression of sexuality. Such an emphasis on "sexuality" as the life force around which neurosis is formed could explain, at least in part, why Freud and the analytic community had such a negative reaction to Ferenczi's paper in Wiesbaden in 1932. Ferenczi's presentation raised very deep questions about the structure and conceptualization of psychoanalytic theory, striking at the prime dogma of the Freudian system in raising a question about the assumption that you can use a sexual vocabulary to talk about children as though they were adults.

The Oedipal conflict arises, in the Freudian system, as a result of the child's inner longing for sexual contact with a parent. Hence, Anna Freud was correct when she said that "giving up the seduction theory would mean to abandon the Oedipus complex . . . In fact, I think there would have been no psychoanalysis afterwards."[19] Indeed, Ferenczi's idea was that the Oedipus complex did not accurately describe the experience of real trauma in instances where children were struggling with the aftereffects of molestation by an adult. At several points in his *Clinical Diary*, Ferenczi suggests that the so-called sexuality of adults in relation to children had more to do with violence than with sexual expression.[20]

Beyond the Confusion of Tongues between adults and children, Ferenczi's approach suggests a rethinking of the category of sexuality generally. In queer novelist Jane DeLynn's fictionalized tale of her sexual experiences, she describes a visit to a dominatrix friend who, while spanking a female client, had a male one kneeling outside her door like a dog. Comments DeLynn, "It was hard to sense the connection between these acts and sex, though I don't know what else you could call it."[21] The implicit question here is a good one. It could be raised also of the child at the breast, as Freud saw it: why not classify this in physiological, affectional, and relational terms, rather than primarily "libidinal" ones? Why not take the sado-masochistic experience as an example of the exercise of power, control, and status, rather than of "sexuality"? The shiftability of such classifications is visible in the movement of the conception of rape, over the last 30 years, from a primarily sexual to a primarily violent and abusive connotation.

To put the same point otherwise: What is the intellectual advantage of collecting these varieties of behavior, as Freud does, under the heading of sexuality? Freud's answer is that it allows us to classify behavior within a unitary framework. "It should be the task of a libido theory of neurotic and psychotic disorders to express all the observed phenomena and the inferred processes in terms of the economics of the libido."[22] In particular, it allowed him to explain psychopathology as a matter of regressions to infantile functioning. But perhaps such a unitary theory, while conceptually economical, does not do justice to the psychological, social, and historical complexities of human experience. Rather than taking games of servitude and domination as forms assumed by fundamental sexual energies, one could open an investigation—of necessity social-historical as well as psychological—into how it comes about that relational structures like sexuality and power can inflect each other in these particular ways.

From this point of view, "sexuality" can be taken, for psychotherapeutic purposes, as a culturally sanctioned classification of a variety of psychological experiences, interwoven with a host of emotional, interpersonal, and intellectual phenomena.[23] This conceptualization differs from the view of sexuality as a drive; it starts from an attempt to understand the child's—or adult's—experience, rather than from positing a biologically rooted essence. As a classification, as a linguistic act, it can seek to impose a conceptual framework on experience, but it can also seek empathically to clarify and develop the subject's self-expression.

The role of language in the construction of sexual experience can be seen in an example of a Confusion of Tongues between a male college teacher and a female student. In the course of a discussion of her academic work, the student approached the teacher, putting her arms around him and making clear her sexual desire for him. Taking this as a confusion on her part, and interpreting her action as a request for affection, he told her, "You don't have to have sex with me to get my attention." The effect of this was striking: she immediately relaxed her body; the sexual embrace was converted into something more like a child's embrace of a parent. After a moment of silence, she confirmed his guess when she said, "Thank you for that." We interpret her acceptance of the teacher's redefinition of the interaction as suggesting that she had suffered from a confusion about her own desire, so that *she experienced her desire for affection as sexuality.* In Foucault's terms, this was an internalization of a socially dominant discourse of sexuality; more specifically, it reflected a particular college subculture that accepted (and even encouraged) student–teacher sexual relationships, which provided a framework consonant with the results of her own intrapsychic struggles.

In understanding this situation, the Confusion of Tongues vocabulary is very helpful. Redefining the experience as a desire for tenderness transformed the encounter from a "sexual" to an "affectionate" one. This example illustrates to what extent the Confusion of Tongues is not just a psychological misapprehension but a physiological experience. That this redefinition of desire was not arbitrary is shown by the student's response to it as allowing her to move in a direction she wished to take. She did not say, "No, I want sex from you, not attention." Apparently, a vocabulary for expressing the desire for parental tenderness was not available to her, other than in the form of sexuality. Once tenderness was offered, and named, the sexuality evaporated into thin air, and never returned, during months of continued meetings.

Ferenczi attempted to theorize such interactions in his analysis of the relations between analyst and analysand in the psychoanalytic situation. Just as he saw the intrusive parent as imposing "passion" (sexuality) on the longings of the child for "tenderness" (affection), so he saw that the analyst can impose his interpretation of "sexuality" on the longings of the analysand for "tenderness" (warmth, responsiveness, support, and empathy). The form of this confusion of tongues, of course, is not that of seduction or emotional demandingness. The analyst acts in a detached, cold manner. Unwilling to form a mutual and emotionally sincere relationship, he or she is engaged in a matter of power and control. In the psychoanalytic interaction as classically conceived, the doctor is in a position *above* the patient, both psychologically and socially unequal. A sick person is submitting to an expert who offers a diagnosis and a cure. Ferenczi did not deny that the analytic relationship was one of unequals, but he conceptualized the relationship as one of unequals who can influence each other toward change. By admitting when he has made a mistake, for instance, the analyst helps to create a situation of trust, which helps the analysand to make use of the analyst's insights.

By calling it a Confusion of Tongues, Ferenczi drew attention to the fact that language is a central medium of power in the psychoanalytic situation. The analyst is invested with the authority to interpret the analysand's experience in terms of his or her theoretical approach. John Forrester has emphasized "the fundamental rule" of psychoanalysis: that the patient should "say whatever comes into your head."[24] What Forrester neglects to mention is the second rule of psychoanalysis, that the analyst reserves the right to tell the analysand the meaning of what has come into his or her head.

Interpretation is one of the main operations by which the analyst maintains power in the relationship. In particular, categorization of the analysand's responses as transference and resistance to interpretations can function as attempts to force the analysand to accept the analyst's way of thinking about the experience. If the former has a very different view of the experience, he or she runs the risk, in the classical situation, of having to submit to the authority of the latter, or else be seen as even more sick or disturbed. After all, if you fervently resist an interpretation intended to make you well, are you not clinging to your sickness? But if you submit to the interpretation, despite its not matching your experience, you are having your reality redefined. So, Ferenczi concluded, if the analysand is being critical of the analyst, wanting a more responsive interaction, the analyst who interprets this (say) as a negative paternal transference reaction is creating a Confusion of Tongues experience for the analysand: a recreation within the psychoanalytic situation of the childhood trauma that brought the analysand to it.

Notes

1 See especially E. Jones, *The Life and Work of Sigmund Freud*, vol. 3 (New York: Basic Books, 1953–1957).

2 See J.E. Gedo, "Ferenczi as the Orthodox Vizier," *Psychoanalytic Inquiry* 17:4 (1997); A.W. Rachman, ed., *A Favorite Son: The Legacy of Sándor Ferenczi* (Northvale, NJ: Jason Aronson, 1997); B. Grünberger, "From the 'Active Technique' to the 'Confusion of Tongues': On Ferenczi's Deviation," in S. Lebovici and D. Widlocher, eds., *Psychoanalysis in France* (New York: International Universities Press, 1980), pp. 127–152; L. Nemes, "Freud and Ferenczi: A Possible Interpretation of Their Relationship," *Contemporary Psychoanalysis* 24:2 (1988), pp. 240–249.

3 A.W. Rachman, "Ferenczi's 'Confusion of Tongues' Theory and the Analysis of the Incest Trauma," *Psychoanalytic Social Work* 7 (Winter 1999).

4 See J. Masson, *The Assault on Truth*.

5 P. Grosskurth, *The Secret Ring: Freud's Inner Circle and the Politics of Psychoanalysis* (New York: Addison-Wesley, 1991).

6 E. Fromm, *Sigmund Freud's Mission* (New York: Harper and Row, 1959).

7 See M. Balint, "The Disagreement Between Freud and Ferenczi and its Repercussions," in *The Basic Fault: Therapeutic Aspects of Regression* (London: Tavistock, 1968).

8 See the discussion in P. Roazen, *Freud and His Followers* (New York: Knopf, 1975).

9 Freud to Ferenczi, December 5, 1931, in E. Falzeder, E. Brabant, and P. Gumperz-Deutsch, eds., *The Correspondence of Sigmund Freud and Sandor Ferenczi*, vol. III (Cambridge: Harvard University Press, 2006), pp. 421–422.

10 Ferenczi to Freud, December 27, 1931, Ibid., pp. 424–425.

11 J. Dupont, "Ferenczi's 'Madness'," *Contemporary Psychoanalysis* 24:2 (1988), p. 255.

12 E.G. Wittenberg, *Presentation of Gyögy Hidas* (New York: William Alanson White Institute, May 1991).

13 S. Freud, "Sándor Ferenczi," *International Journal of Psycho-Analysis* 14:3 (1933).

14 M. Foucault, *The History of Sexuality, vol. I: An Introduction*, trans. R. Hurley (New York: Vintage, 1990), pp. 33, 105.

15 A. Davidson, "Sex and the Emergence of Sexuality," in E. Stein, ed., *Forms of Desire: Sexual Orientation and the Social Constructionist Controversy* (New York: Routledge, 1992), pp. 96, 98.

16 "There may perhaps," Freud wrote, "be an inclination to dispute the possibility of identifying a child's affection and esteem for those who look after him with sexual love. I think, however, that a closer psychological examination may make it possible to establish this identity beyond any doubt" (S. Freud, *Three Essays on the Theory of Sexuality*, ed. and trans. J. Strachey [New York: Basic Books, 1975], p. 89). Why not, when he claims that the "psychoanalytic method" establishes that "most of the so-called bladder disturbances of children younger than four are sexual disturbances: nocturnal enuresis . . . corresponds to a nocturnal emission" (p. 56).

17 Ibid., p. 57.

18 Ibid., pp. 90–91.

19 J. Malcolm, *In the Freud Archives* (New York: Alfred A. Knopf, 1984).

20 J. Dupont, ed., *The Clinical Diary of Sándor Ferenczi*, trans. M. Balint and N.Z. Jackson (Cambridge: Harvard University Press, 1988 [1932]), pp. 79, 173ff.

21 J. DeLynn, *Don Juan in the Village* (New York: Pantheon, 1990), p. 38.

22 S. Freud, *Three Essays*, p. 84.

23 In Davidson's formulation, "Our experience of sexuality is all that there is to sexuality itself, and this experience was decisively and quite recently formed by a set of concepts of categories, among them 'perversion,' and related style of reasoning" ("Sex," p. 122).

24 J. Forrester, *The Seductions of Psychoanalysis: Freud, Lacan, and Derrida* (Cambridge: Cambridge University Press, 1990), p. 35.

4 The Confusion of Tongues Between Freud and Dora

Freud's case of Dora seems to present an especially interesting example of the Confusion of Tongues paradigm that Ferenczi outlined. All of Freud's cases are of interest to students of psychoanalysis, since he used them to illustrate the emergence of the discipline. But his notion that the case of Dora illustrated his Oedipal theory seems, in our view, to be false. It is better taken, we believe, to illustrate his Seduction Theory, the original hypothesis on which psychoanalysis was founded. Ferenczi's ideas about the Confusion of Tongues constitute an expansion of Freud's Seduction Theory, and are more relevant than Freud's to the Dora case. This is one of the first cases to provide a clinical illustration of how sexual trauma can produce emotional disturbance in an individual. By a close examination of Freud's description of this case—his first published case study—we hope to illustrate the efficacy of understanding Dora's disturbance in these terms.

We begin by stating our general thesis, using the terms of Ferenczi's Confusion of Tongues hypothesis: Dora came to her psychoanalysis with Freud wanting "tenderness," but she received "sexuality" or "passion." Freud, therefore, contributed to the Confusion of Tongues experience she was having with adults around her. *He not only tried to convince her that her longing for affection was sexuality but he sexualized their own relationship.* Freud asserted that "the factor of 'transference'" never developed in this "short treatment" (p. 7). If Freud is correct, then, according to his view, a countertransference reaction also did not develop. The treatment was certainly short (the analysis seems to have consisted of three sessions of two hours conducted around 1900; after a break of 15 months, there was one session in March of 1902), but we contend that this seems to have been enough time for an intense transference reaction to develop. As we shall see in more detail, Dora's primary emotional experience of her mother was one of deprivation; of her father, one of narcissistic sexualization of her experience. An intense transference reaction is to be expected in instances

DOI: 10.4324/9781003306559-4

of sexual trauma with an adolescent girl. But Freud's behavior exacerbated the reaction. We are not suggesting that Freud somehow was inherently a negative figure for Dora, but how he responded to her trauma had a negative effect. Dealing with sexual trauma, as Ferenczi demonstrated, mandates a new role for the analyst, one that did not capture Freud's interest. It is perhaps a tribute to the quality and honesty of Freud's writing that his own text makes visible the inadequacy of his understanding and treatment of Dora.

Family Background and Symptoms

It was her father who brought Dora to Freud, with the idea that the doctor, whom he had consulted earlier, should "try and bring her to reason" (p. 42). She was suffering from a number of afflictions diagnosed as hysterical; she also immediately proved to be enmeshed in a complicated set of emotional relationships with her family and friends. At this time sixteen years old (Freud inaccurately gives her age as 18, a matter to which we will return) Dora had been approached sexually by a friend of her father's, Herr K, a man in his forties. She responded by slapping him and complaining to her father. Her father described Dora's "tale of the man's immoral suggestions" as "a phantasy that has forced itself into her mind" (p. 41). That is, he presents the event that precipitated her symptoms as *not a real attempt at "seduction" but as a fantasy on the girl's part.*

Dora's real family name was Bauer. She lived with her mother, father, and her brother, Otto, who later became an important socialist leader. Freud described the father as "the dominating figure in this circle . . . late forties; a large manufacturer in very comfortable circumstances" (p. 12). He had had several severe illnesses by the time Dora was 6 years old: tuberculosis, detached retina, and "a confusional attack, followed by symptoms of paralysis and slight mental disturbances" (p. 13). A friend had persuaded Herr Bauer to go to see Freud after the "confusional attack." Thus, he had himself seen Freud for "hysterical" symptoms. Freud suggests that he diagnosed him as having venereal disease, for which he was successfully treated (p. 13). The father's sister had died of "marasmus" (wasting away, conceivably a mode of anorexia) and his brother was a hypochondriac. According to Freud, Dora inherited a predisposition to hysterical illness from her father's family.

Freud never met Dora's mother. He nevertheless diagnosed her as having "housewife's psychosis," on the basis of the father's and Dora's description of her behavior as "occupied all day long in cleaning the house with its furniture and utensils and in keeping them clean—to such an extent as to make it almost impossible to use or enjoy them" (p. 14). A more sympathetic analyst might have explored the hypothesis that Frau Bauer's obsessive cleaning was an attempt to cleanse herself and the household of the father's venereal disease, because he was a "dirty person," both literally and figuratively. She might well have seen the household as a contaminated place, especially since Dora's father could literally infect his wife. At any rate, simply to ascribe her obsessive housecleaning to "housewife's psychosis" is to deny the reality of her experience of her husband's "dirtiness" and its possible effects on the household. "I was led to imagine her," Freud says, "as an uncultivated woman, and above all as a foolish one, who had concentrated all her interests upon domestic affairs, since her husband's illness and the estrangement to which it led" (p. 20).

Freud's description of the family suggests that there was a fundamental disturbance in the relationship between the mother and daughter: "the relations between the girl and her mother had been unfriendly for years. The daughter looked down on the mother and used to criticize her mercilessly, and she had withdrawn completely from her influence" (p. 20). But Freud does not treat this disturbance seriously. It does not seem to have occurred to him that Dora might have longed for maternal tenderness. In family disputes, the brother apparently took the mother's side; Freud explains this as a manifestation of the son's Oedipal feelings for his mother. But this son, we know, had a highly developed sense of social conscience; why not understand his defense of his mother as an attempt to support her emotionally in the face of her husband's and daughter's rejection?

Dora suffered from severe infections as a child. At the age of 8, she developed a neurotic symptom: dyspnoea (chronic shortness of breath). At 12, she suffered from migraines and attacks of nervous coughing. "At first these two symptoms always appeared together," Freud noted, "but they became separated later and ran different courses" (p. 15). The migraine headaches grew rarer and had disappeared by the time she entered therapy with Freud. Her nervous cough (tussis nervosus) seems to have occurred throughout her childhood. When she came to Freud for treatment the second time, the cough was very evident, lasting for three to five weeks and on occasion for several months: "The most troublesome symptom . . . used to be a complete loss of voice, but the various methods of treatment, including hydrotherapy and the local application of electricity, had produced no result" (p. 15). Freud diagnosed the cough as psychological in origin. (It is conceivable that the loss of voice was related to her complaints about Herr K not having been taken seriously; in other words, as part of the Confusion of Tongues trauma, she lost her voice and the capacity to speak of the trauma.)

Freud describes her as

> a mature young woman of very independent judgment, who had grown accustomed to laugh at the efforts of doctors and in the end to renounce

their hold entirely. . . . Every proposal to consult a new physician aroused her resistance, and it was only her father's authority which induced her to come to me at all.

(p. 16)

It doesn't occur to Freud that he was one more in the line of doctors that her parents had dragged her to. Instead of attributing her resistance, at least in part, to her experience with doctors and her father's authority, Freud assumed the resistance was repressed sexual desires. Freud's interpretation in terms of Dora's unconscious repression of sexuality assumes that there are no other natural responses in an individual's behavior.[1] Freud did not attribute her resistance to his analysis of her problems to a growing sense of independence, which could be seen as a normal developmental trait of an adolescent, nor to the disturbed object-relations she had had with previous doctors. This is a classic example of "blaming the patient."

She described her symptoms when she came to him: "She was in low spirits and an alternation in her character had now become the main feature in her illness. She was clearly satisfied neither with herself nor with her family; her attitude toward her father was unfriendly, and she was on very bad terms with her mother. She tried to avoid social intercourse," instead "attending lectures for women and carrying on more or less serious studies" (p. 16). Apparently, what brought her to therapy was her parents' discovery of a suicide note. After "words" between her and her father, "she had a first attack of loss of consciousness . . . covered by an amnesia" (pp. 16–17). It was then decided that she should see Freud.

Freud suggested that her symptoms of depression, suicidal ideation, migraines, loss of breath, nervous cough, and loss of vitality might all be a kind of malingering. But in fact these symptoms can be more easily understood as reactions to a real event. The event is described as follows: Herr K, a friend of her father's, "had had the audacity to make her a proposal"—that is, proposition her—"while they were on a walk" at a resort the two families were visiting (pp. 18–19). After the incident, Dora told her mother, who in turn told the father. The father, to his credit, confronted Herr K, who denied the incident.

He [Herr K] had then proceeded to throw suspicion upon the girl, saying that he had heard from Frau K that she took no interest in anything but sexual matters, and that she used to read Mantigazza's *Physiology of Love*, and books of that sort in their house on the lake. . . . He had added, that she had been overexcited by such reading and had merely "fancied" the whole scene she had described.

(p. 19)

The father said that this confabulation was at the root of Dora's neurosis:

> I have no doubt that this incident is responsible for Dora's depression
> and irritability and suicidal ideas. She keeps pressing me to break off
> relations with Herr K and more particularly with Frau K, whom she
> used positively to worship. But that I cannot do. For, to begin with,
> I myself believe that Dora's tale of the man's immoral suggestions is a
> phantasy that has forced its way into her mind; and besides, I am bound
> to Frau K by ties of honorable friendship, and I do not wish to cause her
> pain. The poor woman is most unhappy with her husband, of whom,
> by the by, I have no very high opinion. She herself had suffered a great
> deal with her nerves, and I am her only support. With my state of health
> I need scarcely assure you that there is nothing wrong in our relations.
> We are just two poor wretches who give one another what comfort
> we can by an exchange of friendly sympathy. You know already I get
> nothing out of my own wife. Dora, who inherits my obstinacy, cannot
> be moved from her hatred of the Ks. She had her last attack after a con-
> versation in which she again pressed me to break with them. Please try
> and bring her to reason.
>
> (p. 20)

To his credit, Freud did not fully believe Herr Bauer's explanation of Dora's
illness. He accepted Dora's account of her father's affair with Frau K and
her description of K's advances. But he interpreted the effect of these events
on his patient in terms of her supposed Oedipal feelings.

Interpretation and Experience

Dora told Freud of an earlier episode with Herr K which Freud thought of as
an even better example of the Oedipus complex at work. Herr K arranged to
be alone with Dora one afternoon when she was 14 (as Freud tells it; actually she was 12). Herr K "suddenly clasped the girl to him and pressed a
kiss upon her lips" (p. 21). Freud stated that this was "an occasion for sexual
excitement" (p. 22), but Dora "at that moment [had] a violent feeling of disgust . . . and ran to the door" (p. 21). Freud diagnosed her as a hysteric on the
basis of her "disgust reaction." "I should *without question* consider a person
hysterical in whom an occasion for sexual excitement elicited feelings that
were preponderantly or exclusively unpleasurable" (p 22; emphasis added).
Freud calls this a "reversal of affect, one of the most important . . . and difficult problems in the psychology of the neurosis. . . . In this scene . . . the
behavior of this child of fourteen was entirely and completely hysterical"
(pp. 21–22).

It would be reasonable to describe Dora's repulsion as a normal response to a sexual predator. Freud's explanation, however, involves the following tortured argument: When Herr K kissed Dora, she felt his erection, which stimulated her clitoris. She tolerated the excitement and transferred it to her mouth. The mouth was the organ site for the displacement because she had already developed an oral fixation. Freud notes that she was "overindulged in infancy by the habit of sucking for pleasure" (p. 23). The penis is associated with urination, which is in turn associated with defecation. Therefore, the penis is associated with excrement, so that sexual excitement and excrement are closely connected. In this situation, Dora transformed her feeling of excitement into a feeling of disgust.

The least that can be said is that Freud has invented this scenario out of whole cloth. Dora has given no information, according to his own report, indicating that Herr K had an erection, that she felt it against her clitoris, or that she was thereby sexually excited. Freud has made this story up, insisting that it is the basis of an explanation of Dora's experience. In fact, it is a good example of Freud's fanciful theorizing rather than looking at the fundamental interaction between people, as if discerning the psychodynamics of a real relationship was secondary to developing an esoteric symbolic connection.

The Freudian system has always had the aura of being very intellectual, because it emphasizes a high level of abstraction to explain behavior, rather than relying on the data of experience. The phenomenology of immediate experience was not of interest to him. What is actual becomes explanatorily less valuable because it does not have symbolic meaning. He saw the meaning and symbolic value of relations between people as less valuable than intrapsychic phenomena, which he identified with the symbolic pathways whose existence he deduced. For Freud, the actual network of human relationships that existed for Dora and Herr K is less important for explaining Dora's reaction than the chain of associations Freud imagined that led from erection to excrement.

Freud acknowledges that "the forced kissing episode" was a sexual trauma. *But the trauma, in his eyes, is that Dora reacted neurotically to sexual pleasure.* Freud doesn't conceive of the episode as one of the unwanted sexual harassments, intrusive, aggressive, or frightening. He does not conceptualize Dora as being angry, scared, or confused. His emphasis lies on how Dora displaces the sexual excitation that he imagines the episode precipitated. It is not an object-related but a biologically driven experience. It is not a two-person but a one-person experience. The entire emphasis is on how the episode was intrapsychically transformed.

Dora had figured out that her father was having an affair with Frau K: "In [Dora's] mind there was no doubt that what bound her father to this

beautiful woman was a common love-affair" (p. 2). The two families vaca-
tioned together, taking a suite of rooms in common at a hotel. It was normal at the time among the upper-middle class for the man to take separate
rooms from his wife and children. "One day, Frau K had announced that she
could not keep the bedroom which she had up till then shared with one of
her children" (obviously a separate room away from her husband). "A few
days later Dora's father had given up his bedroom" (p. 26) so that he was
also separate from his wife and children. "And they [Frau K and the father]
had moved into new rooms—the end rooms—which were only separated
by the passage, while the rooms they had given up had not offered any such
security against interruption" (p. 26). These rooms seem to have offered less
chance of Frau K and Dora's father being interrupted in their affair. Freud
recognized this situation, in any case a normal sort of marital arrangement
for his class and time, but doesn't acknowledge it as having any meaning
for Dora's experience.

When they returned to town, "her father had visited Frau K at definite
hours, while her husband was at his business" (p. 26). People talked about
the affair. Herr K "complained bitterly" to Dora's mother about it, but not to
Frau K, Dora's father, or Dora, so they maintained an illusion of friendship
even though the affair was known (p. 26).

There was an unusual episode between Dora's father and Frau K: He was
in the woods one day so distraught that he decided to kill himself. Frau K
convinced him to live, he said, for the sake of his family. Dora did not
believe this story, thinking it was an invention to explain why they were
caught in the woods together. Dora may have believed her father wanted to
make love to Frau K, not to commit suicide. Freud linked Dora's disbelief
in her father's suicide attempt with her own suicide attempt, as a disguised
expression of sexual love: "This is the point with her own *pretense at suicide* [italics added], which may thus be regarded as the expression of a longing for a love of the same kind" (p. 26 n. 20). It is Freud's contention that
what you accuse in another you accuse in yourself: "a string of reproaches
against other people leads one to expect the existence of self-reproaches
with the same content" (p. 28). Freud interpreted Dora's suicide attempt not
as connected to any loss of love or nurturance, or to her experience of sexual
abuse, but as a symbolic expression of a desire for sexuality.

Dora gives other evidence of the affair between Frau K and her father.
While the analysis of Dora was going on, Frau K and the father "were in
Vienna, so she told me [Freud is speaking] at that very moment, and she
frequently met her father with Frau K in the street" (p. 27). Herr K, on the
other hand, was clearly preoccupied with Dora at this time of the analysis:
"She also met Herr K very often, and he always used to turn round and look
after her; and once when he had met her out by herself he had followed her a

long way, so as to make sure where she was going and whether she might not have a rendezvous" (p. 27). At no time in Freud's description of these events, of Frau K's affair with Dora's father and Herr K's sexual preoccupation with and harassment of Dora, does he treat the reality of the sexual activities as significant. They are described as if they were secondary events, part of the backdrop to truly important symbolic meanings. Dora's realistic reaction to her father as an adulterer and to Herr K as a lecher is for Freud secondary to her internal sexual strivings. This was Freud's contribution to the story, the transformation of real events into symbolic or intrapsychic events.

Ferenczi was the first to emphasize the object-relations issue in such a triangle, as opposed to the Freudian Oedipal fantasy. Freud chose to ignore the obviously disturbed interaction between these people, which provided a meaningful explanation for Dora's difficulties. Why would one postulate an esoteric concept like "displacement upwards" (from the genitals to the mouth) to explain Dora's disgusted reaction to Herr K, when it would be more parsimonious to say that Dora was reacting to forced sexual contact with an adult? In his understanding of this event, Freud suggests that a man who wants to have sex with a woman defines the experience; the woman ought to get excited and want sex also. If she doesn't, there is something wrong with her. Ferenczi, almost 30 years later (1933), would be able to stay closer to the data. In terms of his Confusion of Tongues theory, Herr K's activity is abusive, an adult forcing a child to view sex as affection (when the child sensed it was aggression). She was looking for affection from Herr K, not having found it with her mother, Frau K, or, now her father, who seemed to be handing her over to Herr K. So when Herr K kissed her in a clearly erotic way it was a betrayal of Dora, who wanted affection, not sexuality. Freud also had a confusion of tongues with Dora, because he defined her reality as sexual.

Freud had difficulty making the distinction between affection and sexuality many times in his life. As we noted earlier, Freud accused Ferenczi of being sexual with his patients in the development of his Relaxation Therapy, when he was being tender and motherly in the attempt to ameliorate the effects of early trauma. On the other hand, Freud did not see the sexuality in his analysis of his daughter Anna, thinking it was only affection.[2] Freud argued that since Herr K was relatively young and good-looking, Dora would have been excited by his kiss. Like Herr K, Freud himself was about 40 years old at this time (see p. 22 fn. 15). But he does not record the idea of his own identification with Herr K.

This is not to say that Freud was unaware of or simply dismissed certain realities in the sexual entanglement of these relationships. For example, he was very much aware that Herr K was romancing Dora and that Herr K and Dora's father were bartering these women:

When she was feeling embittered she used to be overcome by the idea that she had been handed over to Herr K as the price of his tolerating the relations between her father and his wife [Frau K] . . . The two men had of course never made a formal agreement in which she was treated as an object for barter.

(p. 27)

"But as a matter of fact things were in a position in which each of the two men avoided drawing any conclusions from the other's behavior, which would have been awkward for his own plans" (p. 28).

It was possible for Herr K to send Dora flowers every day for a whole year while he was in the neighborhood, to take every opportunity of giving her valuable presents, and to spend all his spare time in her company, without her parents noticing anything in his behavior that was characteristic of lovemaking.

(p. 28)

Freud, however, was at one with the culture of his class and time in finding all this behavior acceptable. He didn't take these facts as reasons for Dora's reaction. It seems no exaggeration to say that for Freud the interpersonal relations in this family are unimportant with respect to the psychodynamics of the case. The assumption that Freud makes that renders the familial interactions unimportant is that Dora wishes to engage in sexual behavior. He assumes that she is repressing her true sexual feelings, and the psychoanalytic method he proposes compels him to attack her defenses, that is, to engage her in a struggle to understand her unconscious sexual wishes. *He does not conceive of the psychoanalytic task as one of tenderness, where the analyst creates an emotional atmosphere of safety, trust, empathy—the opposite of attacking defenses—and acceptance so that the individual would be willing to expose their inner self.* In a tender-minded approach, where empathy predominates, the analyst could investigate as to whether repressed sexuality lurks in the recesses of the analysand's mind, and guard against this assumption being the analyst's confabulation. The empathic method not only creates safety and understanding for the analysand but serves as a check on the analyst's theoretical intrusions.

The same issues arise in Freud's understanding of the relationship between Dora and her governess.

There has been someone in the house who had been anxious at an early age to open her eyes to the nature of her father's relations with Frau K, and to induce her to take sides against her. This was her last governess, an unmarried woman, no longer young, who was well read and of advanced views.

(p. 29)

In a footnote, Freud says of her that she

used to read every sort of book on sexual life and similar subjects, and talk to the girl about them, at the same time asking her quite frankly not to mention their conversations to her parents, as one could never tell what line they might take about them. For some time I looked upon this woman as the source of all Dora's secret knowledge, and perhaps I was not entirely wrong in this.

(p. 29, fn. 1)

Freud is not interested in the relationship between the governess and Dora, which the latter experienced as one of emotional manipulation when the former urged her to demand that her father break off his affair with Frau K. Dora was aware of the governess's motive for talking ill of Frau K:

She might be blind in one direction, but she was sharp sighted enough in the other. She saw the governess was in love with her father . . . . She did not become angry until she observed that she herself was a subject of complete indifference to the governess, whose pretended affection for her was really meant for her father.

(pp. 29–30; pp. 88–91)

In discussing Dora's anger at the governess, Freud suggests that she was angry at a woman for having romantic feelings about her father, forcing it into the Oedipal framework. Furthermore, Freud suggests the anger comes from Dora's own feelings of guilt about her love for Herr K. He does not consider the possibility that the governess's behavior was yet another disappointment in Dora's search for maternal affection. This becomes clear when Dora realizes that the governess is emotionally interested in her father and not in her. As a governess, the woman's special interest is supposed to be in the child, Dora. What is more, the governess had given reason to believe that she was interested in her by paying special attention to the girl.

"What the governess had from time to time been to Dora, Dora had been to Herr K's children." With these words, Freud introduces the idea of Dora's sexual interest in Herr K.

She had been a mother to them, she had taught them, she had gone for walks with them, she had offered them a complete substitute for the slight interest which their own mother showed in them . . . . Herr K and his wife had often talked of getting a divorce; but it never took place . . . . Her preoccupation with his children was evidently a cloak for something else that Dora was anxious to hide from herself and from other people . . . namely, that she had all these years been in love with Herr K.

(p. 30)

Dora denied this at first when Freud suggested it to her, but seemed to acquiesce when he brought up more "evidence" to prove it to her: Despite her complaint about being an object of barter, Dora acquiesced in the relationship with Herr K. Why then did she refuse him at the lake? Freud's explanation is Dora's fear of sex, stemming from childhood masturbation combined with her fear of having inherited her father's syphilis.

Again, in search of evidence, Freud connects Dora's illnesses with Herr K's absences from town, though there is no reason to think that they are connected. This is in turn explained: "it no doubt became necessary to obscure the coincidence between her attacks of illness and the absence of the man she secretly loved, lest its regularity should betray her secret" (p. 32). In discussing Dora's symptoms, Freud states that all hysterical symptoms are combinations of physiological and psychic elements, but he emphasizes the sexual aspect, rather than a relational aspect, of the psychological meaning. Apparently in an attempt to demonstrate the power of his sexual theory he seizes on Dora's nervous cough as a symptom that developed out of a repressed sexual desire. In Freud's interpretation of Dora's illness, her symptoms represent a means to gain her father's attention, "to touch her father's heart and to detach him from Frau K" (46). They are thus also the expression of a sexual fantasy.

Freud sees Dora as seeking her father's sexual attention; he doesn't consider the idea that she might be seeking her mother's emotional attention, or her father's. Illness is a way of extorting affection from those who won't give it: "the motives of illness . . . a means of enticing out its parent's love, and will make use of that means as soon as it has the necessary psychic material at its disposal for producing an illness" (45). This formulation fundamentally proposes a developmental process that *normally* leads to an experience of deprivation. In other words, sharing a parent with another parent (or sibling) naturally leads to pathological behavior. What is missing here is an analysis of the interpersonal experience of deprivation. Freud treats Dora's symptoms not as a response to a pathological situation but as a pathological response to a normal situation.

Freud talked about a "craving for love" as a neurotic trait, an unusual desire, or a "more intense" craving for the parent, which gets joined up with sexuality. He links this craving to seduction in a footnote: "The decisive factor in this connection is no doubt the early appearance of true genital sensations, either spontaneously or as result of seduction or masturbation" (p. 59 n. 1). It is remarkable that he places masturbation and seduction at the same level, equating a two-person with a one-person experience.

The logic of his interpretation of Dora's symptoms is built on Freud's faith in his capacity to interpret the data, rather than on empirical demonstration of the truth of interpretation.

Here are the steps of Freud's interpretation of Dora's symptoms: (1) Speaking to Freud, Dora says that Frau K only loved her father because he was "ein vermogende Mann," a man of means. (2) On the general principle that unconscious meaning is repressed, Freud interprets this statement as meaning the reverse of its manifest content, to wit "ein unvermogende Mann," a man without means, also an impotent man. He leaves out how he arrived at the latent meaning and why the latent meaning is more significant than the manifest one. Even though "unvermogend" can have the meaning of impotent, it is not a word Dora used. "Unvermogend" is actually *Freud's* association. He doesn't stop to ask himself why he is having this association, and what bearing it has on his understanding of Dora's functioning. True, as is often said in relation to the Dora case, Freud had yet to discover the issue of countertransference. But he could have come closer to a two-person psychology if he had paid more attention to what Dora said than to how it fitted into his theory—if he had been more attuned to Dora's subjective experience. (3) Nonetheless, according to Freud, Dora accepted his interpretation: "Dora confirmed this interpretation from her conscious knowledge . . . that her father was impotent" (p. 47). His interpretation was that her nervous cough was due to her preoccupation with "a scene of sexual gratification *per os* [by mouth] between two people" (p. 47). (4) Though he presses her to say the sexual gratification she has in mind is oral sex, Dora doesn't agree. No matter what, Freud insists upon his interpretation. And, according to him, "Dora tacitly accepted this explanation [and] her cough vanished" (p. 48). It is unclear as to what extent Dora actually accepted the interpretation. She may simply have acquiesced to his authority. Freud also acknowledges that the symptom may have disappeared spontaneously.

Discussing her father's relationship with Frau K, Dora observed to Freud that there is more than one way to give sexual pleasure. This led him to imagine Dora fantasizing a man getting oral sex from a woman. But Dora's father was impotent. The data do not suggest fellatio. It is conceivable that Freud was expressing his own fantasy of wanting oral sex with Dora. He sees her as wanting sex with him. He seems strangely insistent on this idea without any real evidence. He seems to need some response from her that he doesn't get. And he seems without noticing it to have transformed the idea of oral as a substitute for the genital sex of which Dora's impotent father is incapable into oral sex performed on the man! This is a confusion of tongues!

Freud's Confusion of Tongues

Freud, rather than Dora, sexualizes the relationship between them. He sees her not as an innocent child but as a pervert, repressing her sexual wishes, because of her hysterical symptoms. By seeing her as a pervert, he feels entitled to say sexual things to her without thinking that he is seducing (traumatizing) her. *Dora* has these ideas and feelings, in her unconscious mind. Freud is only trying to make conscious what is unconscious.

Freud establishes—"to my own satisfaction"—the interpretation by means of his own theorizing, not by testing the hypothesis against the data of Dora's subjective experience or their actual interaction. Freud suggests that Dora was predisposed to oral symptoms because she was a thumb-sucker (p. 44). And Dora is interested in penises, Freud claims, without data from her subjective experience. So she is likely to have a fantasy of putting the penis in her mouth, substituting it for her thumb (breast = thumb = penis). Freud sees eroticism not as part of a relationship, but as a one-person experience with a body part. It is a discharge of energy to satisfy a drive located in Dora.

Freud doesn't try to elicit from Dora why she is so upset. He is so wedded to a one-person psychology that he is actually having an interaction with himself, not Dora. He uses his theory to *uncover* why she is so upset. He doesn't look at what is actually happening between Dora and her father, to discover what may be causing the difficulty. Why is Dora angry with her father? Why is she so obsessed with his affair with Frau K? Freud answers: because she is in love with her father and jealous of Frau K. "The myth of Oedipus is probably to be regarded as a poetical rendering of what is typical in these relations" (p. 56). Why does the Oedipus myth clarify the situation? Oedipus in Sophocles's play has no wish to have sex with his mother, but finds himself trapped in that predicament. The Oedipus myth perhaps allowed Freud to see the child's sexual response to the parent as biologically determined, rather than as a relational experience. At any rate, Freud enjoyed the intellectual interaction with himself as a classically educated person.

Freud uses his own special logic to achieve confirmation of his interpretation. In one instance with Dora, he asserts that she is completely "in love" with her father. But Dora rejects the interpretation, saying, "I don't remember that." In response, Freud uses Dora's association with a female cousin as a confirmation of his Oedipal hypothesis. Given Dora's remembering that her cousin wanted to marry her father, Freud attributed the same desire to her (p. 57). Any denial, according to Freud, actually reinforced the interpretation:

> The "No" uttered by a patient after a repressed thought has been presented to his conscious perception for the first time does no more than register the existence of a repression and its severity; it acts, as it were, as a gauge of the repression's strength . . . . In such cases "No" signifies the desired "Yes."[3]

It is worth noting Freud's recognition of his desire for the "Yes," which he finds even where the analysand says "No." But Freud does not consider a possible relational issue between himself and Dora in her rejection of his interpretation. Instead, Freud would have us believe that a direct rejection can be a confirmation:

> There is another very remarkable and entirely trustworthy form of confirmation from the unconscious, which I had not recognized at the time this was written: namely, an exclamation on the part of the patient of "I didn't think that" or "I didn't think of that". This can be translated point blank into: "Yes, I was unconscious of that."
>
> (p. 50n. 34 [note added in 1923])

This is another variant of the Confusion of Tongues: No again means Yes. The authority is always right, and the analysand's frame of reference is denied. She is not helped to become more confident in her own feelings and thoughts, her own interpretation of reality; instead, she must accept the frame of reference of the other. Built into traditional psychoanalytic thinking is the lack of awareness that insisting on an interpretation of unconscious mechanisms may be a denial of the subjective experience of the analysand. In order for the analysand to be a "good patient," she must deny her own experience and assume the experience of the analyst. This is why an analytic approach based on this tradition is essentially flawed: because it does not take into account the interpersonal relationship or the subjective experience of the analysand.

This use of interpretation is an exercise in power, control, and status over the analysand. The interpretation is not a hypothesis that is used to develop a mutual effort of exploration but an opportunity to create a power struggle, as Freud's words attest: "My powers of interpretation had run dry that day; I let her go on talking, and she suddenly recollected that it was Herr K's birthday too—a fact which I did not neglect to *use against her*" (59; emphasis added). It sounds as though Freud was angry at her and used his interpretation to express his anger. His idea that Dora had sexual longings for her father was not an empathic attempt to discern her subjective experience, but a power play in which Freud is determined to convince her of the efficacy of his idea.

Sex and Symbols

Freud attempts to make a case that Dora is also sexually infatuated with Frau K: "When Dora talked about Frau K, she used to praise her 'adorable white body' in accents more appropriate to a lover than to a defeated rival" (61). This seems another example of Freud's confusion of tongues, his inability to distinguish affection from sexuality. Freud cannot imagine any but a sexual interest on Dora's part. He does not, for instance, consider that Dora might be seeking maternal attention from Frau K and expressing sensual and affectionate, but not sexual feelings toward her.

Similar issues arise in Freud's analysis of a dream of Dora's:

> *A house was on fire. My father was standing beside my bed and woke me up. I dressed myself quickly. Mother wanted to stop and save her jewel case, but father said: I refuse to let myself and my two children be burnt for the sake of your jewel case. We hurried down stairs, and as soon as I was outside I woke up.*

> (p. 64)

Freud doesn't investigate the possibility that this dream may be a reaction to the event of being sexually harassed by Herr K, and her father's failure to protect her, illustrated by the dream statement, "the house is burning down and father doesn't save me." The dream could also be interpreted as Dora's reaction to her mother's narcissism: the mother is more interested in saving her "jewel case" than her children. Instead of focusing on Dora's feelings about her mother, however, Freud aims his interpretation, as usual, at the father. In his interpretation, the dream is the story of a danger, with which her father is associated, and which appears in the night. This will later be connected with Herr K, for, according to Freud, the danger is Dora's sexuality, with which she can only deal by having a relationship with a man:

> The dream confirms once more what I had already told you before you dreamed it—that you are summoning up your old love for your father in order to protect yourself against your love for Herr K. But what do all these efforts show? Not only that you are afraid of Herr K, but that you are still more afraid of yourself and the temptation you feel to

yield to him. In short, these efforts prove once more how deeply you loved him.

(70)

Freud clearly has in mind that the jewel case in the dream is symbolic of a female's genitals. While he tries to convince Dora of this interpretation, she does not accept it (pp. 68–69, 70, 72). This has, as usual, no effect on Freud.

Alan Esterson's *Seductive Mirage*,[4] which examines Freud's work in obsessive detail, finds that the so-called Seduction Theory was developed by dubious means. According to Esterson, in the 15 cases that Freud cites as evidence for the role of childhood seduction in the etiology of neurosis, only one indicated that the patient spontaneously remembered the traumatic moment. In the other 14 cases, Esterson demonstrates, Freud exerted psychological and physical pressure to induce memory recall, in many cases unsuccessfully. From the beginning, Freud had a predilection for proving his theories by getting his patient to fit the theory, rather than by fitting the theory to the experience of the patient. This is certainly true in Dora's case.

Freud's theory of infantile sexuality was a remarkable attempt to conceptualize a sequential development of sexuality in human beings, so that sexual feelings could be understood in relation to a significant history in an individual's development. When sexual issues arose in adulthood, one then had a framework for investigating their origins. But, given Freud's mode of conceptualization, it also spelled the reduction of all actual experiences of sexuality to symbolic manifestations in the child's mind. In its application to Dora, her actual confusion and conflict in dealing with the behavior of the adults around her were reduced to early infantile sexual wishes. The impact of the disturbed behavior of the adults on Dora is seen as less significant than her own fantasizing. The problem then seems to lie in Dora's distortions of the experience, not in the sexual behavior of the adults around her.

Herr Bauer had venereal disease (Freud does not specify its nature), which he got, presumably, from visits with prostitutes. He passed the disease onto his wife, who developed a vaginal discharge, "a catarrh (leucorrhea)," and went to Frazenbad for a cure (p. 67). Dora, Freud says, was also afflicted with the same catarrh. Neither connecting the disease to contamination by the mother or father nor inquiring as to whether the discharge was similar to theirs, Freud assumes that it was of psychological origin. A Victorian in his negative attitude to "self-abuse," he links the discharge to masturbation, so that it becomes a manifestation of Dora's sexuality. Children, according to Freud, masturbate because they get pleasure; when their development leads them to stop the sexual feeling becomes expressed in a hysterical symptom, connected to the end of the Oedipal phase; the cure for hysteria is to transfer the need for sexuality to a suitable mate. (On pp. 71–73 the origin of the problem is located in the unsatisfied sexual desire of the child, who must find satisfaction in one form or another.)

The difficulty is that if Dora's emotional problems are not sexual in origin then Freud is being unempathic and at worst damaging to her by insisting that they are. Freud puts together the determinants of Dora's attacks of coughing and hoarseness (p. 74): Her irritation of the throat is organically determined, "but this is the lowest stratum." This organic site was "susceptible to fixation" because it concerned a part of the body that had for Dora retained to a high degree its erotogenic character. Freud links her thumb-sucking to her mouth as an erotogenic zone, so that throat and mouth are psychologically connected. Dora is involved in a symbolic imitation of her father (he was ill with venereal disease, Dora with a cough). Her illness also represented her relationship with Herr K; it could get better when he was around, worse when he was away. It represented "sexual intercourse with her father by means of Dora's identifying herself with Frau K" (p. 75). Dora's childhood vaginal discharge is linked to "psychological wrappings;" she must have found her own genitals "a source of disgust" (p. 75). In being disgusted by Herr K's sexual advance, she is in actuality symbolically disgusted by her feelings of sexuality (attached to her vaginal discharge and masturbation). Therefore, Herr K's "unwanted sexuality" is beside the point, according to this formulation. Dora is so disgusted with herself that she transfers the disgust onto Herr K. Dora's dream about the fire, correlatively, says on the manifest level that she wishes that her father would save her from Herr K. But in the unconscious mind, more fundamental level, it represents

> the temptation to yield to the man [Herr K] out of gratitude for the love and tenderness he had shown her during the last few years and it may perhaps have revived the memory of the only kiss she had so far had from him.
>
> (p. 77)

Dora wants to sleep with Herr K, but she is afraid to do so. Therefore, she summons up her Oedipal wish to sleep with her father, in order to protect herself from her affection for Herr K.

Freud hypothesized that Dora's father woke her up when she was bed-wetting by kissing her—a rather unusual assumption to make ("and had woken her up, with a kiss perhaps [!], as Herr K may have intended to do" [p. 78]). Her Oedipal wish becomes transformed into a dream: "The infantile, and now unconscious, wish to put her father in the strange man's place had the potency necessary for the formation of a dream" (p. 78). Dora suppressed her wish to have sex with Herr K, because she had learned to associate sex with illness ("her bedwetting, catarrh, and her disgust" [p. 79]). Dora thinks in her conscious mind that Herr K wants to molest her. This is the manifest reality level. But this is characterized in Freud's framework as being a superficial, surface manifestation of a deeper reality. The "real" reason is the unconscious level, where Dora wishes to have sex with Herr K but fears the consequences, because of her own infantile associations of sexuality with illness.

How does Freud know all this, we ask? Feud rests his whole argument on the assumption that a young woman would be flattered by the advances of an older, attractive man (a 14-year-old girl and a man of 40). Dora's discomfort with Herr K's sexual advances can only be a sign of her psychological disturbance. Freud even thinks that Dora's talking to her parents about Herr K's advances to her—which he might more reasonably have seen as an attempt to stop the abuse—is neurotic. "I looked upon her having told her parents about the episode as an action which she had taken when she was already under the influence of a morbid craving for revenge" (p. 87).

Since Freud thought that sexual relations with a man would allow satisfaction of Dora's libido and a cure for her hysteria, he considered Herr K's proposition a healthy resolution of Dora's emotional difficulties. Freud hypothesized that Dora's illness expressed the following sequence of unconscious thoughts (p. 74):

> I am my father's daughter, I have a catarrh, just as he has; he has made me ill, just as he made mother ill. It is from him that I have gotten my evil passions, which are punished by illness.

Freud does not accuse her of evil; he is a man of the Enlightenment. Dora, in his view, developed an illness because she has passions which are natural and need to be satisfied. His message to her is, then: It is because you don't admit to these passions that you are punished by this illness. The first person to whom Dora must admit these passions is Freud.

Freud uses what he calls "symptomatic acts" (p. 68), such as Dora toying with her reticule while lying on the couch, as indications of the truth of this theory connecting her symptoms with masturbation.

> Dora's reticule, which came apart at the top in the usual way, was nothing but a representation of the genitals, and her playing with it, her opening it and putting her finger in it, was an entirely unembarrassed yet unmistakable pantomimic announcement of what she would like to do with them—namely, to masturbate.

(p. 69)

This action was, in his view, doubly symbolic: Freud believed that Dora was exhibiting the desire to recreate the unfulfilled sexual experience (with her father) with him.

Instances of this kind can lead one to believe that Freud had a particular need to see young people as sexual. The stretch that he makes in interpreting Dora's behavior as sexual is very large. Nevertheless, such sexual interpretations became a test of the clinician's capacity to analyze human behavior, as Freud's preoccupation set a standard for psychoanalysis as an interpretive science. His followers came to question their scholarly or intellectual capacity if they failed to see the sexual meaning of a piece of behavior. Not empathic understanding but the discovery of symbolic sexual meaning became standard.

Freud similarly interprets the second dream of Dora in sexual terms:

> *I was walking about in a town which I did not know . . . Then I came into a house where I lived . . . and found a letter from Mother . . . saying that as I had left home without my parents' knowledge she had not wished to write me to say that Father was ill. "Now he is dead, and if you like you can come." I went to the station ["Bahnhof"] . . . I saw the station in front of me and could not reach it . . . Then I was at home . . . The maidservant opened the door to me and replied that Mother and the others were already at the cemetery ["Friedhof"].*
>
> (p. 94)

Freud believed that the unknown town reflected a visit Dora had recently paid to Dresden, where like all nineteenth-century visitors she admired Raphael's Sistine Madonna in the city art museum. She told Freud that

> she remained two hours in front of the Sistine Madonna, wrapped in silent admiration. When I asked her what pleased her so much about the picture she could find no clear answer to make. At last, she said, "The Madonna."
>
> (p. 88; see pp. 95–96, fn. 20, where Freud sees the Madonna as Dora)

Freud focuses on the idea of the Madonna as the virgin mother; he relates this image to sexuality, specifically what he is certain is Dora's wish to be deflowered by a young man. When he learns that she had recently asked her mother where was a box someone had given her, Freud's mind leaps to the question in the dream, "Where is the station?" Since in his mind the box must signify Dora's genitals, the sexual connotation of the dream is confirmed. Freud's interpretation of what he takes to be symbols makes him believe that Dora wanted to lose her virginity. He goes on to outline his idea that Dora's alleged attack of appendicitis was a neurotic symptom of a desire to have a child with Herr K (pp. 91–95). Dora is the Madonna, according to Freud, since she had a hysterical pregnancy (i.e. the appendicitis attack, as Freud interprets it) and is still a virgin.

A few pages later (p. 99), Freud free-associates further. Dora spoke of a *Bahnhof*, and a *Friedhof*, in recounting her dream. These lead Freud to think of *Vorhof* ("forecourt," used in German to mean "labia"); thus the three words serve him as stepping stones to the issue of sexuality in Dora's second dream. Though Dora never mentioned the third of these words, the one that actually has a sexual connotation, Freud takes the words to be symbolic of a "geography of sex" (p. 99). He cleverly associates words given to anatomic parts of the female genitals, known to him as a physician, while acknowledging that even many physicians are not acquainted with the terms. For example, Dora uses the words "nymph" and "woods" in her association to the painting. In Freud's mind, "nymph" becomes "nymphae," an anatomical term for the labia minora, which lie in the background of the "thick wood" of the public hair (p. 99). The logic that makes Dora's use of these terms symbolic of meanings known to an educated physician like Freud is very difficult to follow. (But, as noted earlier, in the Freudian tradition, a clinician's failure to follow such chains of association might demonstrate his or her incapacity as an analyst.) The only connecting link seems to be Freud's assumption that an adolescent driven by sexual curiosity would have read an anatomical text or encyclopedia. There is no reason to assume that Dora had these associations. Rather, Freud seems to be expressing his own sexual associations without identifying them as such. Doing so would have introduced the idea of countertransference. But he was so wedded to his Oedipal interpretation that he could not discuss the subjective experience of the analyst as making a contribution to the experience between analyst and analysand.

Dora's Termination

Dora "opened the third sitting [session] with these words: 'Do you know that I am here for the last time today?'" Freud replied, "How can I know, as you have said nothing to me about it?" (p. 105). In this interchange, Freud shows no concern or empathy regarding Dora's decision to terminate. And although his response sounds defensive and perhaps angry, he says nothing about his own feelings. Dora's response—"Yes, I made up my mind to put up with it until the new year" (the date was December 31)—clearly indicates that she found the analysis unpleasant and suggests that the relationship between them was strained. Freud does not address either of these issues. His words of agreement, which could be seen as empathic, are more likely to have been angry, because they do not come in the context of exploring their relationship: "You know that you are free to stop the treatment at any time. But from today we will go on with our work" (p. 105). Rather than respond to the change in their relationship, which Dora initiated, Freud folds her words into his already constructed theory about her. Once again, he gives the impression that he is only interested in her feelings in so far as they fit his theory.

Here as generally, Freud avoids making his reactions part of the analytic process. Yet one can discern his feelings in the next interchange: "When did you come to this decision?—A fortnight ago, I think.—That sounds just like a maidservant or a governess—a fortnight's warning" (p. 105). Is Freud calling her a servant, who gives two weeks' notice? To suggest that an upper-class girl is acting like a servant would appear to be a hostile remark. In fact, it is Dora who is firing Freud without notice. She had earlier revealed to Freud her lack of respect for her earlier physicians. Freud was being put in their disrespected ranks.

Rather than discussing their relationship, Freud leads her to a discussion of Herr K's relationship with her governess. He suggests that Dora has compared herself to the governess. Because Herr K treated her like a servant, Freud is saying, she acted like a servant. It requires, as so often, a series of interpretations for Freud to demonstrate to her that she identifies with the governess: "To prove to you how deeply impressed you were with the governess's story, let me draw your attention to the repeated occasions on which you have identified yourself with her both in your dream and in your conduct" (pp. 106–7). Like the governess in reality, so Dora in fantasy, according to Freud, longed for a sexual relationship with her father.

Dora made no verbal reaction to Freud's interpretations, which focused on her neurotic Oedipal problems. She neither contradicted him nor agreed with him. Did that indicate a compliant attitude? His interpretation did not move her to continue her analysis. Freud describes Dora's response as follows: "Dora had listened to me without any of her usual contradictions. She seemed to be moved; she said goodbye to me very warmly, with the heartiest wishes for the new year, and came no more" (pp. 108–9). Dora's capacity to remain polite need not be taken to indicate more than that she was a well-brought-up middle-class young woman.

After Dora's termination, Freud spoke with Herr Bauer.

> Her father, who called me two or three times afterwards, assured me that she would come back again, and said it was easy to see that she was eager for the treatment to continue. But it must be confessed that Dora's father was never entirely straightforward. He had given his support to

the treatment so long as he could hope that I should "talk" Dora out of her belief that there was something more than a friendship between him and Frau K. His interest faded when he observed that it was not my intention to bring about that result.

(p. 109)

Freud expresses no need to examine the relationship between himself and Dora to undo—or understand—the premature termination. If her father had sent her back to him, that would have been alright, but on her own, he knew, she "would not come back again" (109).

Freud's frank and honest admission that he was aware that Dora's termination was most likely final indicates an awareness that their relationship was flawed. But he localized the disturbance in her. The patient was flawed. In his view, she had developed a negative parental transference as a result of her neurosis. In Freud's frame of reference, cure was to be effected by interpretation, rather than by examination of the relationship. The more problematic the relationship became, the more he insisted on his interpretations. Freud saw Dora's breaking off the treatment as an act of self-destructive defiance and vengeance. She had become upset at his interpretations, which presumably were undermining her neurotic adaptation. She killed the messenger rather than receiving the message.

The understanding of the Oedipal conflict is a convenience that analysts, following Freud, have developed for their own satisfaction. It allows them to feel that they understand the patient's problem and how to solve it. But analysands do not come to analysis in search of Oedipal interpretations. They come wanting to be understood. It may be that in the course of an analysis an Oedipal interpretation may provide understanding. But understanding is only beneficial in the context of an empathic relationship.

Freud does not seem to have considered the possibility that he was contributing to a negative therapeutic effect by insisting on his interpretations rather than analyzing the difficulties in his relationship with Dora. Instead, he saw the negativity as stemming entirely from her.

Her breaking off so unexpectedly, just when my hopes for a successful termination of the treatment were at their highest, and her thus bringing those hopes to nothing—this was an unmistakable act of vengeance on her part. Her purpose of self-injury also profited by this action.

(p. 109)

Freud was clearly wounded by Dora's premature termination. But neither his own wound (her rejection of him) nor her wound (her unmet need for affection or tenderness) seemed to him to require attention:

No one who, like me, conjures up the most evil of those half-tamed demons that inhabit the human breast, and seeks to wrestle with them, can expect to come through the struggle unscathed. Might I perhaps have kept the girl under my treatment if I myself had acted a part, if I had exaggerated the importance to me of her staying on, and had shown a warm personal interest in her—a course which, even after allowing for my position as her physician, would have been tantamount to providing her with a substitute for the affection the longed for, I do not know.

(p. 109)

Freud, as his words indicate, wanted her to stay in treatment. Yet he chose not to do what he believed would help her to do so. Dora, Freud was clearly aware, wanted tenderness. But he chose to give her cool, "objective" interpretation. He assumed the pose of a scientist, not of an empathic healer.

One can easily feel empathy for Dora as one reads Freud's account of her struggles. Freud was able to evoke empathy in the reader, so one could assume he had an empathic response to Dora. *Why then not give her tenderness, if this is what she sought?* There are several levels of explanation. First, not her need for tenderness but her Oedipal issues were seen as central to cure. Freud's focus was on Dora's relationships with the men in this story, not her difficult relationship with her mother. This skewed the issues in a sexual direction, especially because he interpreted the affectionate relationship between a girl and her father as sexual. Freud consistently interpreted her desire for affection as a sexual wish, imagining a homosexual desire for Frau K or an identification with the Madonna as impregnated woman.

Second, Freud saw himself as a scientist. He envisioned reacting to Dora with tenderness as a nonprofessional manipulation:

I have contented myself with practicing the humbler arts of psychology. In spite of every theoretical interest and of every endeavor to be of assistance as a physician, I keep the fact in mind that there must be some limits set to the extent to which psychological influence may be used, and I respect as one of these limits the patient's own will and understanding.

(p. 101)

Freud seems to indicate the importance of not influencing the patient by suggestion or aggressive interpretation—though this is what in practice he did. What he does not seem to understand is that by not responding empathically he created a psychological distance from the person in analysis. (This was one of the chief differences between Ferenczi and Freud: the one saw himself as a healer, the other as a theory builder.) He felt he could not tamper with the "resistance" by giving Dora what she wanted. It was more important to prove his theory was correct than to help Dora.

The two wounded parties in this therapeutic encounter were unable to resolve their difficulties or fulfill their needs. They were caught up in a Confusion of Tongues. Dora could not speak of her longing for affection or tenderness from Freud. She was aware of needing this from her mother and Frau K, but could not express the need to have it fulfilled by her analyst. There was something missing in the transferential relationship, so that the analysand could not express this kind of wish. She, the child in the relationship, was urged to believe her desires were sexual, though she felt they were affectionate. Her reality, because she was emotionally vulnerable, was distorted by her experience with Freud. She told him she needed affection; he replied that she was sexually disturbed. It was actually a sign of her strength that she left.

Freud likewise could not speak of his disappointment in Dora's premature termination or engage in any dialogue which dealt with the disturbances in their relationship. From his point of view, the patient was acting out her unresolved Oedipal transference (that is, by leaving Freud, Dora acted out her Oedipally produced anger toward Herr K). Her behavior toward Freud was purely transferential. The actual relationship with Freud functioned only as a signifier for her Oedipal situation. Freud did not view transference as being reenacted in the analytic situation. If Freud had been more attuned to Dora's subjectivity than to theory building, he might have discovered this.

Freud relates in a postscript that Dora returned to his office 15 months later and asked to resume the treatment to deal with a recurrence of her symptoms. She had run into Herr K in the street when he had been struck by a carriage. She had "another attack of aphonia" (lost her voice) for six weeks and developed a "right-sided facial neuralgia" (p. 121). She described to Freud a remarkable event that shows her emotional courage: she elicited from Frau K an admission of her affair with Dora's father, and she got Herr K to admit his—previously denied—sexual misconduct at the lake, and "brought the news of her vindication home to her father" (p. 121). Freud does not depict himself as responding in any way to her courage or to the accuracy of her earlier reports of Herr K's sexual abuse. Instead, he uses the material she brings him to validate his Oedipal theory.

We speculate that Dora's ability to confront the Ks, come and report to Freud about it, and later get married testifies more to her ability to emancipate herself from Freud along with the other adults around her than to the accuracy of Freud's interpretations. She may have used the negative transferential experience of her analysis with Freud to emancipate herself from him, her father, and Herr K. Freud, in any case, rejected her attempt to return to his care. "Dora came to see me again," he writes, "to finish her story and to ask for help once more. One glance at her face, however, was enough to tell me that she was not in earnest over her request" (pp. 120–1).

Freud, we believe, was clearly confused about Dora's return to analysis when he said, "I do not know what kind of help she wanted from me, but I promised to forgive her for having deprived me of the satisfaction of affording her a far more radical cure for her trouble" (p. 122). It was Freud's one-person psychology that prevented him from inquiring as to what Dora wanted, when it was unclear to him. The analyst analyzes the patient's "resistance," not the interaction between them. Freud had offered help, in the form of analyzing Dora's issues as a function of her unresolved sexuality. She did not accept this. He interpreted the lack of acceptance as resistance, an inability to deal with her anger and give up her neurosis (the neurotic refusal to be cured). His final gesture of help was to forgive her.

He said, "I do not know what kind of help she wanted from me." In his frame of reference, if you offer a patient the opportunity to be analyzed, that is, to understand that their difficulties are a function of their unresolved Oedipal issues, and they don't accept this help, you must conclude they are "unanalyzable." Even if they return, as Dora did, if they do not say, "I came back to accept your interpretations and struggle with my resistances," they remain unanalyzable.

Freud interpreted the facial neuralgia as a displacement of Dora's feelings of guilt for hitting Herr K after his harassment of her at the lake. But she also, he thinks, feels guilty about rejecting Freud, onto whom she had transferred her feelings about Herr K. So Freud represents her neuralgia as symptomatic of her sexual desire for him. He forgives her for rejecting him (by prematurely terminating) so she does not have to punish herself anymore for rejecting him, by developing facial neuralgia. Freud here exhibits a narcissistic preoccupation with the analyst, though ignoring the analyst's contribution to the relationship with the analysand.

Freud seems to have no interest in exploring why she has returned. He did not feel he was unempathic or unresponsive to her need for tenderness. However, a greater demonstration of caring for Dora would break a methodological rule of treatment. He wouldn't be acting like a scientist or doctor. Since he felt that her reaction to him (need for tenderness) emanated from her sexual conflict (her unresolved Oedipal issues), responding tenderly would be tantamount to responding sexually. Therefore, responding tenderly would create a potential sexual experience for the patient, which would be both unprofessional and not therapeutic.

Freud's Prohibition on Showing Affection

Freud's theory of transference underlies a theoretical rationale and a clinical uneasiness in dealing with affectionate interactions. The theoretical rationale comes from his belief that "sexuality is the key to the problem of the psychoneuroses and of the neuroses in general" (p. 105). Freud could not differentiate between affection and sexuality. To show affection, for him, is to behave sexually, and so to go beyond the boundaries of professional behavior. This also explains Freud's reaction to Ferenczi 30 years later, in the "kissing letter," discussed in the previous chapter. Freud wrote to Ferenczi admonishing him not to pursue therapeutic touching of his patients, because he thought of this as the first step toward sexuality.

Dora, as Freud saw it, was transferring her affection from Herr K to her analyst. Freud reasoned: if I respond to her affection, I will be playing the same role as Herr K. It would be better for me to remain a scientist and not respond. Here is another dimension of Freud's Confusion of Tongues with Dora. Dora sexualized their relationship, he thought. So if he responds affectionately, it would be taken as sexuality. The adult interprets the child's affection as sexuality, treating the child as incapable of distinguishing affection from sexuality. What is more, it is the child, not the adult, who is the seducer. It is *Dora's* sexual transference to Freud that is the problem:

> Psychoanalytic treatment does not create transferences, it merely brings them to light, like so many other hidden psychical factors. The only difference is this—that spontaneously a patient will only call up affectionate and friendly transferences to help towards his recovery; if they cannot be called up, he feels the physician is "antipathetic" to him, and breaks away from him as fast as possible and without having been influenced by him. In psychoanalysis, on the other hand, since the play of motives is different, all the patient's tendencies, including hostile ones, are aroused; they are then turned to account for the purposes of the analysis by being made conscious, and in this way the transference is constantly being destroyed. Transference, which seems ordained to be the greatest obstacle to psychoanalysis, becomes its most powerful ally, if its presence can be detected each time and explained to the patient.
>
> (p. 117)

Freud here utilizes his theory of transference to indicate that the patient is to blame for the sexualization of the relationship.

It is not just sexuality as a factor motivating an individual in human interactions; the individual's neurosis *is* the sexuality. So when Dora leaves analysis, according to Freud, she is acting out her rage at what she experiences as Herr K's rejection of her. Her behavior—so Freud sees it—has nothing to do with anything that Freud has done in their clinical interaction. The analyst believes he is functioning in a sterile surgical field, free of any contaminants, because the focus is on the internal manifestations of the patient's transferences. In this conceptualization, the emotional and interpersonal factors in the clinical interaction within the therapeutic dyad are seen as irrelevant. Freud believed Herr K was acting "normally." He was expressing sexual desire for a desirable young woman. Dora reacted neurotically when she rejected Herr K. Herr K behaved like a gentleman and left her alone, but Dora was angry at Herr K for leaving her alone. She displaced this anger onto Freud, according to the transference theory, and left analysis, preventing him from curing her.

Here, we have an exaggerated but literal form of the Confusion of Tongues. There is almost nothing that Dora can do that Freud would not interpret as sexual. Dora becomes frustrated, confused, and angry because her acts are misinterpreted. Freud, like the other adults in Dora's life, denies the truth of her experience. Dora's father denies that he is having an affair with Frau K. Herr K denies he made a sexual advance to Dora at the lake. Freud insists that Dora is sexually interested in her father, Herr K, and Freud; he even interprets Dora's affection for or interest in Frau K as homosexual desire. Given all this, Dora's "active rebellion"—leaving the analysis—can be viewed not only as a typical adolescent rebellion against an authority figure but also as an attempt to cure the Confusion of Tongues, by maintaining a sense of her own reality and self-cohesion in the face of an authority's attempt to dictate to her.

Another aspect of Freud's analysis of Dora is the fact that he can interpret her behavior only in terms of his theory of infantile sexuality. He doesn't have a framework for viewing Dora's subjective experience. He can ask, for example, why the idea of marrying Herr K is problematic for Dora. He has no framework for viewing her rejection of this idea as a positive attempt at self-actualization. Freud realized that something was wrong between them, but he attributed it to a reaction by Dora:

> I did not succeed in mastering the transference in good time. Owing to the readiness with which Dora put one part of the pathogenic material at my disposal during the treatment, I neglected the precaution of looking out for the first signs of transference, which was being prepared in connection with another part of the same material—a part of which I was in ignorance.
>
> (p. 118)

Why was Freud not able to discover the two-person psychology that Ferenczi initiated later on?[5] Freud actually had ample opportunity to make such a discovery, both in the Dora case and in earlier cases detailed in the *Studies in Hysteria*. If we follow the Freudian tradition, the answer is: if analysis is necessary to come to an awareness of your deepest conflicts, then Freud lacked a personal analysis. Because he was unwilling to have an analysis—either formally or in the form of a mutual experience such as both Jung and Ferenczi offered on different occasions—he had an unanalyzed transference.[6]

The problem with Freud's later discovery of the countertransference reaction is that it did not alter his view of the psychoanalytic encounter as a one-person experience. He viewed the countertransference reaction as a hindrance to the analytic process, something to get rid of as soon as possible so that the analysis can continue (see the next chapter for further discussion of this issue). From a two-person point of view, in contrast, the counter-transference appears as a part of the analytic process, to be understood and integrated into the analytic encounter. It is thus not only that Freud failed to have an analysis but also something was flawed in his conception of analysis, with its image of the physician as observer rather than as participant in a two-person system.

> In this way the transference took me unawares, and, because of the unknown quantity in me, which reminded Dora of Herr K, she took her revenge on me as she wanted to take her revenge on him, and deserted me as she believed herself to have been deceived and deserted by him.
>
> (p. 118)

Freud takes "some detail in our relations," the "unknown quantity," as an unanalyzable fact. It cannot be understood. He does not inquire into what the detail is, and discuss it. Why wouldn't an analyst ask an analysand, "What is the detail in our relations which troubles you?" Freud's theory already has an answer to this question. Dora is transferring her anger toward Herr K onto Freud. He therefore knows what the problem is: it is Dora's transference. So there is no need to explore their relationship. What is needed is for Dora to share his understanding.

When she doesn't share it and prematurely terminates, Freud hints at feeling hurt and rejected: "No one who, like me, conjures up the most evil of those half-tamed demons that inhabit the human breast and seeks to wrestle with them can expect to come through the struggle unscathed." Freud appears to express anger in turning Dora away when she returned for treatment. Remarkably, he speaks of a promise "to forgive her for having deprived me of the satisfaction of affording her a far more radical cure for her troubles." It seems obvious that he is the angry one; though he says that "I do not know what sort of help she wanted from me," he rejected her as a patient rather than explore modes of helping other than Oedipal interpretation.

That this was not the only possible response was shown when, first, Ferenczi and later Hans Kohut had the wisdom to accept the analysand's plea for empathic understanding, with the effect of positively changing the course of treatment.[7] Ferenczi's treatment of Elizabeth Severn is a landmark in psychoanalysis because for the first time the analyst's response to the analysand was the focus of the analytic process. Ferenczi made the effort to attune himself to his analysand's complaints about his functioning as the source of the so-called resistance. He developed what became known as mutual analysis, in which the analysand was to inform him about his functioning in the same way in which he informed her about hers. It is worth quoting from Ferenczi's description *in extenso*:

> There was a point over which we came to be at loggerheads. I maintained firmly that she ought to hate me . . . She resolutely denied this, yet these denials at times were so ferocious that they always betrayed feelings of hatred. For her part, she maintained that she sensed feelings of hate in me, and began saying that her analysis would never make any progress until I allowed her to analyze those hidden feelings in me. I resisted this for approximately a year, but then I decided to make this sacrifice.
>
> To my enormous surprise, I had to concede that the patient was right in many respects. I had retained from my childhood a specific anxiety with regard to strong female figures of her kind. I found and continue to find [sympathetic] those women who idolize me, who submit to my ideas and my peculiarities; women of her type, on the other hand, fill me with terror and provoke in me the obstinacy and hatred of my childhood years. The emotional superperformance, particularly the exaggerated friendliness, is identical with the feelings of the same kind which I had for my mother.
>
> Mutual analysis . . . gave me an opportunity to vent my antipathy. Curiously, this had a tranquilizing effect on the patient, who felt vindicated; once I had openly admitted the limitations of my capacity, she even began to reduce her demands on me. As a further consequence of this manifest "circulus benignis," I really find her less disagreeable now . . . My interest in the details of the analytical material and my ability to deal with them—which previously seemed paralyzed—improved significantly. I must even confess that I am beginning to be aware of the beneficial influence of this liberation from anxiety in relation to other

patients as well, and thus I am becoming, not only for this patient, but also for the others, altogether a better analyst.[8]

Kohut expanded on Ferenczi's discovery. Writing about his treatment of Miss F., who rejected his interpretation of her associations, he acknowledged that for "a prolonged period . . . I was inclined to argue with the patient about the correctness of my interpretations and to suspect the presence of stubborn hidden resistances."[9] Like Ferenczi, he was finally able to accept her frame of reference and to treat her reaction not as "resistance" but as a "plea for empathy," which made it possible to think about the relationship, thus enabling the analysis to proceed. Kohut presented the admirable example of someone who, hampered by the traditional approach, was able to emancipate himself. Both Ferenczi and Kohut were able to switch their allegiance from Freud to their analysands. Freud, in contrast, could not shift his primary allegiance to understanding Dora from her point of view; instead, he insisted on understanding her from the standpoint of his emerging Oedipal theory. This is why the analysis was a failure.

Notes

1 This was well captured by a joke at the height of psychoanalysis's popularity in the United States in the 1950s: Two psychoanalysts meet; when one says, "How are you?" the other wonders, "What did he mean by that?"
2 See A. Rachman, *Psychoanalysis and Society's Neglect of Sexual Abuse of Children and Adults: Reassessing Freud's Original Theory of Sexual Abuse and Trauma* (London: Routledge, 2022).
3 S. Freud, *Three Essays*, p. 51.
4 A. Esterson, *Seductive Mirage: An Exploration of the Work of Sigmund Freud* (Chicago: Open Court, 1998).
5 See A. Rachman, *Elizabeth Severn, the Evil Genius of Psychoanalysis* (New York: Routledge, 2018).
6 See A. Rachmann, *Sándor Ferenczi: Psychotherapist of Tenderness and Passion* (Northvale, NJ: Jason Aronson, 1997).
7 See H. Kohut, "The Psychoanalytic Treatment of Narcissistic Personality Disorders: Outline of a Systematic Approach," in *The Psychoanalytic Study of the Child* (New York: International Universities Press, 1968), pp. 23, 86–113; H. Kohut, *The Analysis of the Self* (New York: International Universities Press, 1971).
8 Sándor Ferenczi, *Clinical Diary*, pp. 98–99.
9 H. Kohut, "The Psychoanalytic Treatment of Narcissistic Personality Disorders," pp. 503–504.

5　From "Transference" to "Mutuality"

We believe that this reanalysis of the case of Dora adds material for a revision of the concepts of transference and countertransference that has already been underway in psychoanalysis for some time. The traditional concepts of transference and countertransference are inadequate because they conceptualize the analysand as construing the analyst as if he or she were a parent rather than viewing the relationship between them as having parental characteristics. The traditional concept of transference drags with it an outlook that is no longer adequate for viewing the analytic encounter as a relationship. It reduces transference and countertransference in the analytic relationship to the Oedipal conflict.

Freud mentions countertransference—the factor that would make analysis a relational experience—as early as 1909, but he viewed it as something to get rid of (see his 1910 letter to Jung),[1] as something shameful, not as something to use. His intellect allowed him to discover countertransference but, beyond his idea of himself as a scientist and an objective observer, his personality did not allow him to use his discovery to alter his therapeutic method. In order for his method to incorporate countertransference, Freud would have had to become intimately connected to his own traumas and be willing to explore them; his unwillingness is suggested by his rejection of Ferenczi's offer of analysis. (Marianne Krüll has noted in particular that Freud could not explore his sexual trauma with his nursemaid because of the family prohibition on keeping secrets.)[2]

Often, defenses of Freud's clinical behavior with Dora suggest that he did not do as well as he might have because he had not yet discovered countertransference, an idea Freud himself expressed in the 1927 edition of *Dora*. From this point of view, Freud's problem was a lack of technical knowledge. Hannah Decker's article, "Freud's Dora Case," provides an interesting example of this tendency because Decker is a feminist sympathetic to Dora's struggles, who goes so far as to see Freud as engaging

DOI: 10.4324/9781003306559-5

in a form of sexual harassment in the course of her analysis. And yet she does not discuss Dora's psychological predicament in terms of her actual relationship with Freud. Instead, she depicts each as caught up in transference vis-à-vis the other. "Freud," she says, "failed to help Dora substantially because he was limited by his incomplete knowledge" (p. 114), not understanding his countertransference to his patient.[3] It seems more accurate to say that he was limited by his inability to explore his own traumas and their consequences for his intellectual and emotional development as well as his relationships with others.

The traditional notion is that transference and countertransference are disturbances in the relationship, needing to be interpreted genetically to cure the disturbance. The analysand is distorting the relationship; the analyst is responding neurotically to this transference reaction. From our point of view, both analyst and analysand are creating the experience between them, in reaction to and relation to each other. This is why it is not the saying of words, giving correct interpretations based on reconstruction of the past, that is curative, but the nature of the here-and-now relationship in which the words are said.

Dora terminated prematurely, we have suggested, because the nature of the actual relationship between her and Freud (as opposed to the imaginary relationship he imputed to her) was not addressed. As we have stated repeatedly, if Freud had not been so intent on proving the efficacy of the Oedipal theory, he would have been able to use the Dora case to develop the beginnings of a relational view of psychoanalysis. The kernel of a relational view is embedded in Freud's description of his interaction with Dora. In fact, she was trying to co-create a relationship with him by telling him what she needed. Freud chose to ignore her needs, because he wasn't interested in that aspect of the analytic encounter.

Ferenczi developed Freud's notion of the countertransference reaction into the far-reaching notion of a countertransference analysis. Rather than viewing countertransference as a reaction interfering with the analytic process, he viewed it as the analyst's contribution to the process. Such a development naturally unfolds from his two-person psychology, that is, the analytic encounter is construed as a relational experience between the analyst and analysand where both parties contribute their personal, intellectual, and interpersonal data.

Ferenczi's desire to examine the analyst's contribution to the psychoanalytic situation was fueled not only by intellectual curiosity but by his identity as a healer. As he became more and more immersed in the psychoanalysis of his "difficult cases," he was forced to examine his own functioning. Part of his clinical genius is that he went beyond the traditional formulation when a difficulty arose in the analysis, by not invoking a resistance interpretation. If you do not "blame the patient" for the difficulty by interpreting their psychopathology, you are left with a need to examine the dynamics between analyst and analysand. Ferenczi had the courage to scrupulously examine his own functioning as it contributed to difficulties in the interactions between himself and his analysands. He did so not to abuse the privilege of analyzing himself for the sake of his own self-indulgence but to contribute to the analysand's recovery.

For example, in the analysis of Elizabeth Severn, chronicled in the *Clinical Diary*, when Ferenczi reveals his own difficulties in emotionally relating to her and women generally, he is doing so to repair his relationship with her as well as to contribute to repairing Severn's view of men, shaped by a severely traumatic history with a sadistic father. Had Ferenczi insisted on describing her difficulties with himself as resistance, she might have experienced this as the act of a new "abusive father." She had already sensed something in Ferenczi's response to her that was interfering with their relationship. By admitting his contribution to their problem, he showed his disinclination to blame her and willingness to examine himself as a basis for improving that relationship.

Countertransference analysis, from this point of view, is the ongoing examination of the analyst's functioning—intellectual, clinical, and personal—as it enters the analysand's experience. It must continue throughout the analysis, for without it we would be back in the traditionally conceived situation of the analyst analyzing the analysand without the idea of a relational experience. It is thus not a hindrance but an aid to the analytic process. One does not get rid of one's countertransference but becomes increasingly attuned to it, and so more able to use one's reactions to contribute to the understanding of the process. The goal is not the elimination of countertransference reactions but the understanding of them and the creative use of them in changing the analyst's functioning in the analytic encounter.

We give an example of an analysand, similar in age and personality to Dora. A 14-year-old girl, she came from a disadvantaged family, with an absent father and a hardworking mother who was often out of the home. At the end of each session, she took to giving the analyst a kiss on the cheek. How was he to react to this? One possibility in deciding how to deal with it was to scrutinize his own reaction to the kiss, looking for evidence of sexual stimulation. He found none, and this suggested the nonsexual character of the kiss on her part as well. The teenager came from a Latino background, where physical demonstrations of affection are natural between adolescents and adults. The analyst himself (A.R.), coming from a European background, never stopped kissing his daughter and son hello and goodbye through their teenage years, a practice that began in childhood and continued into their adulthood. This is the framework in which he allowed this teenager to kiss him goodbye.

This was a potentially erotic transferential–countertransferential interaction. Had he had erotic feelings, accepting these kisses would have been to encourage some unexamined erotic experience between the two of them. Note that this would not have been a matter of seductive behavior on her part, but of an experience between the two. As it was, however, the kisses could be accepted and responded to as filial, as answering a need for parenting. This experience of 30 years ago has stayed with A.R. because it helped him understand how a physical gesture, such as touching or kissing, by an analysand isn't necessarily sexual. On the basis of his analytic training, he would have had a negative reaction to this gesture. But being able to view it as something occurring between the two of them, and examining his own participation, freed him to elasticize the analytic situation, construing it in terms of affection, rather than eroticism.

Decker explains the classical concept of transference: "The analyst must not take these 'transference neuroses' as reality."[4] Of course, there is a sense in which this is right: the analyst should not react as a lover. But it leaves out the fact that the transference reaction is a current reality, and not just an appearance of a past desire. If the analyst just says, "These feelings, you know, aren't really about me," something that's actually going on is not being attended to. In the classical version, either the analyst becomes caught up in countertransference and responds inappropriately, or else claims that the analysand's feeling has nothing to do with him at all. But the truth lies elsewhere: there is an actual emotional experience involving the two of them in which he should not engage inappropriately.

What does Ferenczi's understanding of the Confusion of Tongues dynamic lead to, in this context? The most fundamental issue in the cure of the Confusion is emotional honesty, clarity of communication, and a literal interpretation of behavior. In its simplest terms, we need to "say what we mean and mean what we say." Curing the Confusion of Tongues requires both members of the therapeutic dyad to strive to express honestly what they feel, communicating it in an empathic way. For example, an analysand says, "You seem irritated with me." The traditional analyst might reply, "No, this may be an example of your transference of your fear of an angry father." But if the analyst is in fact irritated or frustrated, or angry, it is essential that he or she acknowledges that aspect of the analysand's perception which is accurate. Not doing so would mean not encouraging the experience of reality. So the analyst might reply, "Yes, I am feeling irritated. Let's discuss why I might be feeling irritated with you." This gives a mandate to explore and express, in a judicious way (so as not to retraumatize the analysand), the interpersonal meaning of the interaction. What is called for is self-awareness in relation to the other person, open, honest, and non-defensive communication for the purpose of creating a more self-determined, self-defined experience.

Speech cannot be isolated from the rest of the experience. A significant idea of the Confusion of Tongues paradigm is that a trauma is created when a child is maltreated by an adult and, because of the adult's superior power, is unable to speak of the trauma. The child therefore becomes tongue-tied, submerging their feelings and splitting off the experience from intellectual and emotional awareness. In this way, he or she loses the ability to communicate the traumatic experience in speech. Silent suffering becomes the characteristic response to the trauma. The adult abuser who wishes to change must also undergo a transformation from not being able to speak, from being frightened to speak, to finding the courage to speak about it. He or she has lost the capacity to communicate about this in language, because he or she wants to remain silent about the abusing behavior. So what is created is a conspiracy of silence, one person's silence reinforcing the other's. Language is split off from the traumatic experience (in fact, the child is often threatened, sometimes physically, with an injunction not to speak). Because the person cannot speak of the trauma, the trauma becomes localized in the person's soma, whether in specific organs or body parts. We can speak of somatic memory: There are portions of the individual's body that store the memory of the event without the capacity to verbalize it. Eventually, the somatically stored memories and the feelings connected to them need to become part of a verbal communicative process for the cure to take place.

Speaking about the trauma returns the abused person to awareness of what happened, who did it to him or her, where it happened, and what he or she felt. It is a creative process that counters the continuation of denial, detachment, and dissociation. This is a transformation of the Freudian "Talking Cure." In Freud's system, the speech of the analysand provides data for the analytic scientist's interpretation. In Ferenczi's reconception of the matter, the analysand's capacity to speak and communicate is part of the curative process. The somatic memories need to be connected to speech, to create an emotional insight. The uncovering of the memories can encourage a reconnection between the event and the feelings, which now exist in an adult. This adult is getting help with reexperiencing and understanding what happened, so that the mechanisms of childhood adaptation to trauma are not reinforced. Instead, the trauma must be reexperienced from a more developed, less fragile sense of self, less under the influence of an adult authority, with the support of the therapeutic partner. Here speech plays a new role, not to repress but to explore the experience, to aid in its interiorization and revision.

Being allowed to speak about being hurt, rejected, and abused is in fact a fundamental need—the need to share one's feelings with a significant other. People also need to be affirmed in their feelings. The most fundamental human need is to be confirmed in one's feelings by the person one has those feelings about. Speech is so important in the experience of trauma because it is central to specifically human life. Language is the medium developed by human beings for expressing an open-ended set of meanings, and for making an open-ended set of experiences available for reflection. We know that one of the most disturbing experiences a person can have occurs when individuals are not allowed to speak to one another. For example, putting a prisoner in isolation is considered one of the most stringent punishments. We see this also in the history of feral children—a child reared in isolation does not fully develop human qualities.[5] Being a child is a vulnerable condition for the Confusion of Tongues, because parents are in a position to define reality.

This is why specificity to the analysand is important, why generalization is not good enough—because the adaptation to trauma creates a dissociative experience. Such an experience splits off the feelings, the thoughts, and the remembrance of the events into separate fragments as a way to master the disturbance of the event, or to reduce its disturbing effect. In order to develop mastery as an adult over a childhood trauma, one needs to reconnect these fragments through language into a coherent phenomenological whole. This can only occur if one goes over the original experience with whatever specificity the person can bring to the encounter, recreating the experience and reconnecting it to feelings and thoughts.

It was Ferenczi's idea, derived from the analytic tradition well established in Freud's original writings, that the reason the child's "sexual experience" with the parent becomes traumatic is that the child is unable to metabolize the experience through verbal interaction. (There are, of course, other aspects: betrayal, intrusion, sadism, etc.) If the child's ego is overwhelmed by the experience with a parent, and there is no avenue to fully express the feelings, thoughts, and behaviors to another human being—peer or parent—it forms a secondary traumatization. Being tongue-tied, as Ferenczi characterized not being able to speak of the trauma, interferes with personality development. The child's not being able to speak solidifies its dependence on the abusing person. The child loses a sense of self; it loses power, a grip on reality, and self-esteem, because it places itself in the hands of the abusing parent as the arbiter of reality and deciphering the event. Without speech, one cannot represent the situation and is dependent on the representations furnished by others. Speech equals self-definition, autonomy, a way in which an infant first begins to separate from the mother. When the "I" is no longer a "we," it begins to define the child's capacity to have separate feelings, separate thoughts, and separate behavioral events. Becoming tongue-tied is like returning to the preverbal stage of development.

There is also a nonverbal aspect of this matter, the atmosphere, evoked by "body language," that facilitates speech. Use of touch, feeling, and pictures, bringing into play the full range of human activity, helps recall and eventually verbalization. Ferenczi observed the behavior of analysands as they were lying on the couch[6] and he also experimented with variations in the analyst's behavior. The introduction of these matters into the analytic situation had a positive effect on the freeing up of symptoms. This history indicates how the body stores experiences when it becomes tongue-tied.

To achieve full expression and be able to analyze the feelings, one needs to verbalize them. Psychoanalysis gives credence to the notion that speech in humans is a fundamental curative experience. Unfortunately, the early psychoanalysts relied too heavily on direct verbal interaction, even when the analysand has difficulty speaking. Ironically, the classical method encouraged a "tongue-tied" analyst, who was to speak minimally, and often not at all. Just as Ferenczi loosened the speech of the analyst, it was his idea that when people have difficulty speaking—that is, become tongue-tied—nonverbal means provide alternative methods to help the body remember and to free up the person's ability to speak. This was part of the effort to undo the Confusion of Tongues. Ferenczi's flexibility allowed him to consider the full range of human activity as forms of communication.

To take an example: Alan, an analysand of AWR, was asked to speak freely and as specifically as he could about all the issues on his mind. For the first time in his life, he felt free to speak about the anal matters with which he was fascinated. This reflected the analyst's acceptance that his concern had some meaningful origin, and that it was based on a legitimate feeling. The analyst strove to communicate this by creating an empathic atmosphere in which Alan could talk freely and not be judged. This enabled him to find his voice concerning a childhood trauma.

One day he said that standing by the elevator to leave after a session during which he talked about how everyone in his large family seemed to be concerned with anal matters—one brother buggering another, a sister playing anally with her son—he felt a warm sensation in his buttocks. Thus, the analytic experience opened him to both verbal and nonverbal experiences that he could then speak about. He then had a dream about having anal intercourse with his 5-year-old son. Although beside himself with shame and anxiety he was still able to report the dream—nothing was being left unsaid. He felt that the dream indicated a wish to have intercourse with his son. The analyst, working from a Ferenczian perspective, thought that it might be an indication of a trauma that occurred to Alan around the age of 5. Discussing the dream from the vantage point of a young boy assaulted by a father, the mystery began to be resolved. In this session or the next, Alan remembered the traumatic event. He brought in some strawberries, and offered the analyst some, who accepted them. He then said that he was beginning to remember that the child in the dream was himself and that the father was his father, and that he was beginning to have fragmentary memories of intercourse with his father near an outhouse on their farm, smelling a nearby strawberry bush.

This example indicates the value of helping analysands recover their voice—their somatic-emotional memory—so that they can speak of their trauma. For example, by not viewing the dream as an indication of transference—as a desire perhaps to be abused by the analyst—but as the residue of a real experience, the focus of the analytic session was moved from fantasy to reality.[7]

When is recollection real? This has become an important and contested issue with the rise of so-called repressed memory therapies associated with the excavation of purported sexual abuse. There is evidence that pseudo-memories can be induced; on the other hand, we now know that Freud's original Seduction Theory was not in fact based on memories produced by his patients but on interpretations that he had to belabor them into accepting. At the very least, the analyst must be careful to work on recall from the subjective experience of the individual, using his or her thoughts and feelings, and not imposing the analyst's own ideas. The analyst must not be overly invested in the recall. In fact, the implanted memory is itself a Confusion of Tongues phenomenon, the imposition on the analysand of the analyst's wishes. So the very practice of overcoming the Confusion of Tongues is a prophylaxis against false memory syndrome.

In the case of Alan, he developed his memories on the basis of his own experiences, the analyst being careful not to suggest interpretations but attempting to facilitate the exploration of fragments of memory that came to him. In another case, B., a woman with a life-long history of avoidance of sexual relations with men, brought forth material pointing to incestuous trauma. She was, however, uninterested in following it up. She told the analyst, "You are so interested in analyzing sexual trauma, you believe that everyone has that issue." She was so clearly distanced from the possibility that she had suffered sexual trauma, and so unwilling to examine it, that to do so would have failed to respect her subjective experience. It would have been the same error that Freud made with Dora. It is a person's right not to explore any aspect of their functioning, if he or she does not wish to do so, even if an unexplored, traumatic aspect of the past negatively influences his or her contemporary behavior. The person's statement that he or she is willing to live with his or her dysfunction needs to be respected.

Ferenczi's deconstruction of the psychoanalytic process creates a new atmosphere that favors democratic and mutual interaction.[8] Ferenczi deconstructed the psychoanalytic process by writing a new text for clinical interaction between analyst and analysand. There was a shift from an analyst-centered to a mutually constructed dialogue and process. The Confusion of Tongues paradigm, which gave new meaning to the individual's experience in the parent–child relationship, had implications for the analyst–analysand dyad as well. Retraumatization—that is, the individual reexperiencing aspects of the childhood Confusion of Tongues trauma—was seen to occur in the clinical interaction of the psychoanalytical situation. In the Oedipal view of transference, meaning is created from the analysand's projection onto the analyst of his or her perception of and feelings about parental authority, colored by childhood neurosis. New meaning was available when the text of the psychoanalytic situation was conceptualized as an experience of mutual analytic partners, if you will, constructing the narrative of the analysis together.[9]

Notes

1 W. McGuire, ed., *The Freud/Jung Letters*, trans. R. Manheim and R.F.C. Hull (Princeton: Princeton University Press, 1974).

2 M. Krüll, *Freud and His Father* (New York: Norton, 1986). For further discussion of Freud's childhood sexual abuse, see A. Rachman, *Psychoanalysis and Society: Neglect of the Sexual Abuse of Children, Youth, and Adults: Readdressing Freud's Original Theory of Sexual Abuse and Trauma* (London: Routledge, 2021).

3 H. Decker, "Freud's Dora Case in Perspective: The Medical Treatment of Hysteria in Austria at the Turn of the Century," in T. Gelfand and J. Kerr, eds., *Freud and the History of Psychoanalysis* (New York: Routledge, 1992).

4 Ibid., p. 109.

5 See R.B. Rachman and A.W. Rachman, "The Feral Child in America, Myth and Reality," unpublished paper, 1982.

6 See Sándor Ferenczi, "Technical Difficulties in the Analysis of a Case of Hysteria: Including Observations on Laral Forms of Onanism and Onanistic Equivalents," in J. Rickman, ed., *Further Contributions to the Theory and Technique of Psycho-Analysis*, vol. II (New York: Brunner/Masel, 1980 [1919]), pp. 189–197.

7 See A. Rachman, "The Literal Interpretation of Dreams," in *The Psychotherapy of Difficult Cases* (Madison, CT: Psychosocial Press, 2002).

8 See A.W. Rachman, "Beyond Neutrality: The Curative Function of Analyst Self-Disclosure in the Analytic Situation," in J. Reppen, M.A. Schulman, and J. Tucker, eds., *Way Beyond Freud: Postmodern Psychoanalysis Evaluated* (London: Open Gate Press, 2002).

9 See A.W. Rachman, *Psychotherapy of Difficult Cases* (Madison, CT: Psychosocial Press, 2002).

6 Curing the Confusion of Tongues

As we have indicated in our reanalysis of Freud's clinical interaction with Dora, the Confusion of Tongues created between them originated in a discrepancy between the emotional, interpersonal, and communicative experiences of two people with unequal amounts of power. Freud tried to impose his experience on Dora. On the other hand, Dora, we hypothesize, had a rather different experience. She did attempt to convey her experience to Freud. And as we have shown in Chapter 4, Freud did hear Dora's need for tenderness, but chose to withhold an empathic response on the basis of his theoretical mandate to interpret Oedipal material. It is this kind of discrepancy between the expressed or inferred subjective experience of the analysand and the analyst's unempathic response to it that activates a Confusion of Tongues trauma in the psychoanalytic situation. This Confusion of Tongues between analyst and analysand is a retraumatization, a replay of the original childhood experience with an unempathic adult.

Ferenczi's theory was not only an attempt to understand the psychodynamics but also to delineate the curative factors in the Confusion of Tongues. First, let us outline what Ferenczi suggested are the fundamentals of cure for the Confusion of Tongues trauma. Then we will apply these fundamentals to Freud's analysis of Dora.

A fundamental aspect of cure is emotional honesty. In the clinical interaction between analyst and analysand, both parties must strive for authenticity, that is, to "say what they mean" and "mean what they say." The analyst encourages the analysand to become more aware of his or her feelings through accurate and empathetic understanding of the individual's subjective experience. In response to the analyst's empathy, the analysand becomes more aware of his or her emotional experience.

Second, the analyst actively encourages the analysand to express his or her feelings in an open and direct way. We take an illustration of this point from an incident in an analytic group session: A group member was encouraged to begin the session, because she never initiated interaction.

DOI: 10.4324/9781003306559-6

The therapist and the other members of the group agreed that this would be a meaningful new direction for her, because her lack of open expression had created an emotional distance among them. As things developed, it became clear to all that she was having a great deal of difficulty in freely expressing herself. When the therapist suggested that she seemed defiant, he was attempting not just to interpret her behavior (nor to criticize it) but to encourage her to be honest about her state of feeling. Since the suggestion was a function of empathic attunement, she readily accepted the interpretation, saying, "You're right. I feel like I don't want to give to you or to the group." Of course, by saying that, she was giving. This led to more: She admitted her wish to defy demands from authorities and her fear of hurt if she revealed her feelings; she ended the session in tears. In a following individual session, she said that she thought this interaction was very helpful, and recounted a dream that she interpreted as being about emotional tenderness and responsiveness. Had the analysand rejected the interpretation, it would not have been pursued. The point was to offer not just interpretation but the emotional support, empathy, and insight that the analyst can provide to help the analysand find the courage to be emotionally honest. It works insofar as there is emotional attunement.

Third, developing an egalitarian encounter in the psychoanalytic situation is essential to cure the Confusion of Tongues. In the therapeutic encounter, the analyst's behavior is under scrutiny as well as the analysand's. It was Ferenczi who made the groundbreaking discovery that analyst's self-disclosure is curative of a Confusion of Tongues experience.[1]

Freud's activity was a function of his theoretical framework. This form of activity was not helpful for Dora, since she rejected the interpretations and the process did not lead to her being more emotionally expressive or self-disclosing. His form of interpretation is what has been characterized, by Kohut, for example, as "experience distant" clinical observation of the analysand's behavior and intervention based on the analyst's understanding of the meaning of that behavior. In contrast, Kohut talked about "experience near" observation, an attempt to discern the subjective frame of reference of the analysand, offering an empathic intervention—in Ferenczi's terms, to develop a mutual understanding of the experience.[2]

The danger is, of course, the use of such techniques for emotional manipulation. Here, the therapist must rely on what we might call an "empathic compass," the analyst's ongoing "hovering attention" to the interaction between himself and the analysand, attuned to the impact his interventions are having on the individual. If the person is responding negatively, for example, then the relationship needs to be readjusted, for instance, by inquiring what impact the intervention had on the analysand. This should lead to self-scrutiny of the analyst's behavior.

"Relaxation" was both a concept and an attitude that Ferenczi used in order to designate a significant change in the psychoanalytic encounter. At first glance, relaxation may seem to be an unscientific term to refer to a therapeutic process. But in actuality the term captures the change in emotional and interpersonal experience that Ferenczi created. By "relaxation," he meant: a decided shift from interpretation to empathy; from blaming the patient through the concept of resistance to scrutiny of the analyst's activity; from a sterile field and neutral analyst to encouraging analyst's self-disclosure; from a one-person experience focused on the analysand to a two-person experience focusing on mutual analysis; and from the exercise of power, control, and status to the creation of an egalitarian relationship.[3]

The psychoanalytic situation was classically understood as a formal and traditionally authoritative relationship between a patient and a doctor who identifies an illness and prescribes a cure. Freud was emotional, but did not admit to his emotions. And the analysand's feelings, evoked by Freud, were not allowed into the process, except in the framework of the analyst's interpretations. Being cognitive without being emotionally connected to the person is not helpful. For example, Freud's account of his relationship with Dora indicates that he had emotional reactions to her, but this affective component of the relationship was not included in the analysis.

Ferenczi, in contrast, believed that the patient should be encouraged to be a partner in the analytic process. He actively sought the help of the analysand in creating the analytic treatment. Enlivened and dramatic reliving of experience, rather than an intellectual discussion and analysis of it, produced change grounded in emotional insight. In this enlivened format, actual change could occur within the clinical interaction, which could then be metabolized in the relationship between analyst and analysand.

Self-disclosure, instead of analyst neutrality, encouraged a mutual and egalitarian interaction which allowed the analysand to experience a "new beginning"[4] with a "reparative parental figure."[5] Ferenczi realized that "admitting mistakes" in the psychoanalytic interaction was the way in which a therapist authority could take responsibility for difficulties that arose in the interaction. By being emotionally honest, the analyst creates a positive alternative to the double-bind neurotic parental communication of childhood, where parental culpability was denied. The experience of childhood created a Confusion of Tongues because the parent did not admit to the emotional content of his or her actions that were disturbing the child. By not being emotionally honest, the parent stimulates a sense of confusion, forcing the child to question his or her sense of reality.

The best test of the analyst's capacity to engage in an egalitarian encounter is when an analysand raises an issue about his or her behavior. For example, trauma survivors will suggest that the analyst is expressing anger that is not being acknowledged. In the Freudian as well as many other therapeutic traditions, the analyst interprets the need for self-disclosure, rather than responding with disclosure. But in the Ferenczian framework, an attempt would be made to engage the analysand in a clinical interaction where analyst's self-disclosure would be judiciously offered. So the Ferenczian analyst might say, "I was not aware that I was angry, but let's explore what you heard me say or do that led you to feel that way, and I will try to examine my functioning." This discussion might lead the analyst to reveal that the analysand was correct in observing his or her anger, and the impact that it had on the individual's experience. (This does not preclude analyzing genetic or transferential components of the relationship.) The analyst must of course practice "judicious self-disclosure"[6]—that is, reveal only aspects of the emotional reaction that would be therapeutically helpful in curing the retraumatization experience. Analysands want and need the analyst to demonstrate that he or she is aware of, and willing to acknowledge, the need for a "responsive parent." They do not want an "intrusive parent" who reveals depths of intense anger or rage. Such an expression of emotion on the part of the analyst would be narcissistic and retraumatizing rather than curative.

Ferenczi observed that when he admitted to "mistakes"—that is, to his empathic failures—and explored his contribution to them, a remarkable clinical event occurred. Rather than become frightened, distant, or uncommunicative, as he had been taught in the Freudian tradition would happen, trauma survivors greeted his disclosures with a positive response. They were grateful that he had admitted to and disclosed his contribution to the retraumatization.[7]

Emotional honesty, as exemplified by judicious self-disclosure, is curative of the Confusion of Tongues trauma in several important ways. A new form of communication and interaction is created where there is an egalitarian and two-person experience rather than an analyst-dominated therapy. The analysand does not feel compelled to accept the analyst's version of the reality in the psychoanalytical situation. Rather, he or she can be helped to own up to his or her own version of reality. What is more, the analysand's version of reality will help shape the analyst's perceptions. Both members of the therapeutic dyad will co-create reality in the psychoanalytic situation.

Being able to express one's emotions honestly is relevant to the clinical behavior of both analysand and analyst. For the former, to freely and honestly express emotional feelings, psychological issues, or reactions to the experience with the analyst, it is essential that a safe, trusting, and egalitarian atmosphere be created. It is only through the genuine attitude of the analyst who stimulates emotional experience through an enlivened, active, and, at times, dramatic encounter, that the analysand can be willing to chance free emotional expression.

As has been mentioned, the crucible for emotional honesty occurs in the moments when the analysand "challenges" the analyst to confront his or her own emotionality. Ferenczi's work clearly demonstrated that analysands who suffered intense and debilitating trauma during childhood, due to abuse or unempathic parenting, have a special need for emotional honesty. But this is a general human need, certainly shared by all analysands.

The analyst's willingness to struggle with and scrutinize his or her own emotional functioning is essential. It is only through "the analysis of the analyst," as Ferenczi labeled it, that an analytic encounter focusing on the emotional interaction between the parties can become genuinely therapeutic.[8] Ferenczi believed that the analyst should spend as much time and energy analyzing himself or herself as is necessary to meet the needs of creating an emotionally honest relationship. To pursue a course of analytic self-scrutiny, the analyst must adhere to a theoretical frame of reference that allows for clinical flexibility and responsiveness.[9] We believe Ferenczi's Confusion of Tongues theory provides such a vehicle. We also believe that any frame of reference that incorporates a relational perspective, emphasizing empathy, flexibility, responsiveness, two-person psychology, and analyst self-examination will also be helpful.[10]

How might all these have worked in Dora's case? We offer a clinical fantasy: an imagined interaction between Dora and an analyst willing to attune to the subjective experience of the analysand.

DORA: You have been hurting me, not helping me. That's why I want to stop these sessions.

ANALYST: Well, I'm sorry if I hurt you. I didn't mean to do so. Tell me how I've hurt you.

DORA: You keep insisting on telling me that I'm really attracted to Herr K! It makes me feel bad that you won't believe me.

ANALYST: I regret that my interpretations are hurting you. I want to understand what's bothering you, and I seem to have become so captivated with my theory about it that I haven't been listening enough to you. Tell me more fully how I tried to get you to believe something that you thought wasn't true.

DORA: I tried to tell you that I had a problem with my mother, but you always insisted that I talk about my father.

ANALYST: Maybe you're right about that—I did have the notion that your father was the most important part of your difficulties. Perhaps I was mistaken.

DORA: I'm not saying that I don't have problems with my father, but you don't seem to want to talk about my relationship with my mother. I'm really mad that my mother is so wrapped up in herself.

ANALYST: I think you're right. It was too important for me to prove my theory about your father to hear what you said about your mother. So let's talk about your mother.

Dora's desire to prematurely terminate her analysis was based, as we said earlier, upon her feeling that Freud was not empathically attuned to her need for tenderness. In our little clinical fantasy, the analyst took a step toward such attunement so that he or she could help her focus on this need. When someone wants to leave analysis prematurely, the fundamental issue is to understand the need for separation, without trying to convince the person to stay. In other words, can you formulate a response that relates to the need to separate and reduces the anxiety that has produced it? We are assuming that Dora wanted to leave because she felt traumatized by Freud's intrusive sexual interpretations of her behavior. Our imaginary analyst has to try to reduce his or her own anxiety about the loss of the analysand. Analysts have difficulty letting go of people who want to separate from them. If the person needs to go, they may return only if you help them understand why they are going. We too often see termination as an end point rather than as a part of the process of someone's struggling with the relationship. Dora apparently needed time to reduce the traumatic effect of an imposing male authority upon her and to metabolize the reparative experience of the termination. Understanding this might have helped her to return.

For the real Dora, the story was traumatic rather than reparative. But we, who are living over a hundred years later, do not need to be confined by Freud's example. Dora can help us understand how a young person can struggle to overcome their traumas and gain self-definition in the face of authorities who don't fully understand them. This book pays tribute to youth who too often face negative authority but find their own way. We see Dora as a heroine. She stood up to Freud, as well as to the adults who had traumatized her. She did not kill herself, or accept their definition of what she should think and do. We salute her capacity to define her own reality.

One of the unexplored issues in the Freud–Dora story is the nature of adolescent–adult relationships. Freud's behavior with Dora can be understood as a function of a traditional adult authority exercising power and control over an adolescent.[11] As we have pointed out repeatedly, this exercise of power was most clearly illustrated in the vigorous intrusive attempts Freud made to interpret Dora's so-called Oedipus complex. Dora never had an opportunity to establish a more egalitarian relationship with Freud. Freud was typical of the men of his time, who viewed adolescents more as children, in need of adult control and guidance, than as people becoming adults themselves.

This extended to Freud's feeling that Dora should be *grateful* for Herr K's sexual interest. Thus he urged her to respond to Herr K sexually and to marry him, advice driven by a man's view of what a woman should do. He never explored with Dora her own reactions to Herr K's advances. He didn't encourage her to express her negative feelings about Herr K, her father, or himself, which would have aided the establishment of a more empathic attunement to her frame of reference and a more democratic interchange.

Erik Erikson was a pivotal figure in the history of analytic interest in the Freud–Dora case, as it was he who first discussed the developmental task of adolescence as a crucial element of the relationship between the two. In essence, Erikson helped us see that Freud did not have a theory or a method for understanding and treating an adolescent in trouble. Erikson contributed an understanding of how an adolescent like Dora needed to solve identity problems, about which Freud was oblivious. We feel that Ferenczi's frame of reference adds to Erikson's understanding of how an adolescent like Dora could be better treated. Our understanding of the Confusion of Tongues trauma between Freud and Dora suggests that Freud heightened the issues of power, control, and status, rather than diminishing them. The essence of therapeutic contact between an adolescent and an adult is the capacity to function as a "tender authority figure" (what Ferenczi called a "tender mother transference"). The analyst tries to become aware of and respond to the needs of the adolescent without imposing his or her will. This means focusing on empathy.

For example, instead of heightening the issue of authority, the therapist can share authority, by taking the adolescent's ideas seriously as an integral part of the treatment. When Dora suggested that the relationship with her mother was insufficient, Freud dismissed this suggestion by ignoring it, as though Dora had no understanding of her own condition. In fact, she may have had a greater understanding of what was troubling her than Freud, but was frustrated in trying to explain it to him. Instead of trying to tell Dora what was wrong with her, Freud needed to invite Dora to tell him what she was struggling with.

This issue is particularly important in dealing with adolescents, because one of the fundamental problems between adults and adolescents is that adults are afraid to hear what adolescents have to say, and don't help them find their voice. Of crucial importance in the psychotherapy of adolescents is helping young people to develop the idea that they too can be authorities, above all on their own lives, feeling that they have power, control, and status in a relationship with an adult authority.

Instead, Freud treated Dora like a child who needed to obey him to get better. The irony is that she probably got better when she defied him and left. In Dora's so-called premature termination, she found her voice, in essence saying, "I don't have to take this anymore. I can be free of this oppressive authority." This was, one could say, a partial resolution of the Confusion of Tongues trauma. She did not continue to suffer an emotionally abusive experience with Freud. According to Freud, Dora identified him with her father as an object of Oedipal fantasy. It is more reasonable to think of her as experiencing the two men as similar in their authoritarian and manipulative treatment of her. In her defiance of Freud, then, she could work through some of her problems with her father's authority.

With adolescents, in distinction from adult analysands, there is generally another adult in the picture: the parent or parents (or other adult authority) who bring the child to therapy. In Dora's case, it was her father, we remember, who brought her to Freud with the request that he "bring her to reason." Freud's initial response to Dora was encouraging: he accepted her account of family relationships rather than her father's. Yet he concluded by suggesting that she bow to the adults' will, accepting Herr K as a lover in return for her father's access to Frau K. Freud, like her father, thought she must be "brought to reason," and even that this should involve her acceptance of Herr K as a mate—exactly what her father had, consciously or unconsciously, wished her to do.

In such a situation, the analyst's fundamental task should be to engage the adolescent in dialogue, so that he or she can best understand the adolescent's point of view. Not only is the adolescent's point of view as essential in the process of therapeutic change as any other analysand's, but often the therapist needs to become an advocate for the young person with the parent, helping the latter understand the child's frame of reference. He or she may have to help the adolescent assert himself or herself, to give voice to their frame of reference to understand it themselves and convey it to their parents and other adult authorities.

We believe that there is often a fundamental Confusion of Tongues between adults and adolescents as a result of the inequality of power between them. Adults often attempt to exercise dominance over adolescents. Although this is not a relationship between equals, the adult should attempt to convey in the very setting of limits an empathic understanding of the adolescent's needs, giving the latter an opportunity to voice objections and when appropriate changing the limits. Adult behavior should not be ruled by a narcissistic need to dominate but by a flexible responsiveness to adolescent needs. The other side of this is the child's desire for limit setting as an aspect of being taken care of.

Freud saw children as savages needing to be tamed. The importance of the castration complex as the key to maturation in his theory shows how deeply set in Freud's thought was the nineteenth-century idea that terror is necessary for the transformation of an animal into a human being. Another way of putting this is to say that Freud saw trauma as a necessary part of the normal process of maturation. In his view, the way in which a child is socialized, and gives up their incestuous longing for the opposite-sex parent, is through the fear of castration. The threat of mutilation and annihilation is then normalized as a part of a child's personality development. In this, Freud shows himself to be a man of the later nineteenth century, sharing with other great thinkers of the period—Darwin and Nietzsche come to mind—a conception of life as a violent struggle.

The Freudian emphasis on trauma as reality has promoted the notion among analysts that childhood and adolescence are periods of darkness, and necessarily so. The emphasis is then on what kinds of pathologies emerge as results of trauma-as-reality. In contrast, understanding trauma as catastrophe can highlight the child's or adolescent's capacity to cope, not just his or her experience as an unwitting victim. In the story of his relationship with Dora, Freud at no point says to her, "How wonderful that you never gave in to all those people pressuring you. How strong and healthy you are to have resisted the pressures of these adults and to try to understand reality on your own terms, true to your experience." But how useful this would have been to her—and how true.

Returning thus to our subject, Freud's view of Dora was completely influenced by his notion that Dora suffered a normative crisis: when Herr K tried to molest her and she felt revulsion, she was exhibiting the Oedipus complex. The trauma she suffered was to be expected. (If she weren't so involved in her Oedipal interaction with her father, she wouldn't have reacted with fright and disgust.) What is so striking about Ferenczi's formulation, in contrast, is that he recognized that trauma is a pathological event in human behavior. When it occurs, it indicates that something has gone astray in the object relations within the family setting. The contrast between Freud's normalization of trauma and Ferenczi's conception of trauma as catastrophe is a profound reconceptualization of human reality and personality development.

Ferenczi's Confusion of Tongues formulation, therefore, is a significant alternative theory of human interaction, because it removes trauma from normality and places it as an overwhelming and disturbing experience with negative consequences. This has implications for the understanding of therapy, which instead of being the working through or repetition of trauma, becomes the effort to provide an alternative experience. At the deepest level, it opens up the question of the nature of the relation between parent and child, and between adults and children generally, as opposed to the Freudian idea that trauma is inevitable. What are the social preconditions for the experiences that modern society came to think of as natural?

A fundamental element in the modern relationship between parents and children is the survival of the medieval idea that parents own their children, that children are chattel. Father and later mother therefore can shape the child's behavior to their will, and it is even their job to do so. And the parents have all the power, status, and control. Parents feel that they have the right to impose their ideas and values on their children and restrict their behavior, as justification for proper child-rearing practices, without taking into account the impact of their behavior on the child. It is the child's job to make the best of the circumstances in which they find themselves. Often parents don't consider that they have to provide better circumstances.

What has been termed the child-centered home is also, paradoxically, an example of this phenomenon: It is based on the parent's need to treat a child as though it were a peer, or to assuage their guilt about being overbearing. This is an example of the failure to provide guidelines and limits, which leads to treating the child as a buddy of the parent. This is the imposition on children of the idea that they are adults and that there should be no inequality in the relation between adults and children. It is important to recognize that there is inequality in power, status, and control between adults and children, in virtue of differences in age, experience, and formal status designation, but one ought not to exacerbate these issues in order to manipulate behavior. Actually, one should be mindful of the inequality and function empathically, bearing it in mind, so as not to traumatize the child. The occurrence of control, manipulation, and the absence of limits are both traumatic.

From Freud's point of view, the case history of Dora illustrated at once the natural course of human development from childhood to maturity, marked by trauma, and the analytic experience as the uncovering of this natural course as a basis for understanding and mastering it. The analysand must learn to accept a vision of life as involving a conflict between desires and social power relations, adapting the former to the reality defined by the latter. Drawing on Ferenczi's insights, we have attempted to sketch an alternative picture: one in which childhood experience with adults need not be traumatic, a possibility practically realized in the therapeutic experience, in which an empathic relationship can be constructed and explored.

Notes

1 Sándor Ferenczi, "The Elasticity of Psychoanalytic Technique," in M. Balint, ed., *Final Contributions to the Theory and Technique of Psychoanalysis*, vol. III (New York: Bruno Mazel, 1980), pp. 87–102.

2 H. Kohut, *How Does Analysis Cure?* (Chicago: University of Chicago Press, 1984).

3 See Sándor Ferenczi, "The Principle of Relaxation and Neo-Catharsis," *Final Contributions* III (1930), pp. 108–125; Sándor Ferenczi, "Child Analysis in the

Analysis of Adults," *Final Contributions* (1931), pp. 126–142; J. Dupont, *The Clinical Diary*; Sándor Ferenczi, "The Confusion of Tongues Between Adults and Children."

4 M. Balint, "Character Analysis and New Beginning," in *Primary Love and Psychoanalytic Technique* (London: Hogarth Press, 1985), pp. 157–164.

5 A.W. Rachman, *Psychotherapy of "Difficult Cases": Flexibility and Responsiveness in Contemporary Practice* (Madison, CT: Psychosocial Press, 2002).

6 A.W. Rachman, "Judicious Self-Disclosure by the Analyst," *International Forum of Psychoanalysis* 7 (1998), pp. 263–269.

7 Sándor Ferenczi, "The Elasticity of Psychoanalytic Technique," pp. 87–102.

8 Sándor Ferenczi, "Child Analysis in the Analysis of Adults," pp. 126–142.

9 A.W. Rachman, *Psychotherapy of Difficult Cases*.

10 See A.W. Rachman, "The Confusion of Tongues Theory: Ferenczi's Legacy to Psychoanalysis," in A. Haynal and E. Falzeder, eds. *A Hundred Years of Psychoanalysis* (London: Karnac Books, 1994); A.W. Rachman and C. Mucci, *A Confusion of Tongues Theory of Trauma: A Relational, Neurobiological Perspective* (London: Routledge, 2022).

11 See A.W. Rachman, "Principles of Clinical Interaction in Adolescent Group Psychotherapy," *Issues in Group Psychotherapy* 5:1 (2001), pp. 39–75.

Index